The Medicine Society

Paul Scriven

The Medicine Society

Paul Scriven

Michigan State University Press
East Lansing
1992

All Michigan State University Press books are produced on paper which meets the requirements of American National Standard of Information Sciences—Permanence of paper for printed materials ANSI Z23.48-1984

Michigan State University Press
East Lansing, Michigan 48823-5202

Printed in the United States of America

00 99 98 97 96 95 94 93 92 1 2 3 4 5 6 7 8 9 10

Library of Congress Cataloging-in-Publication Data
Scriven, Paul
   The medicine society / Paul Scriven
      p   . cm.
   Includes bibliographical references and index.
   ISBN 0-87013-315-2
   1. Drug Abuse—United States   2. Drug Abuse—United States
3. Narcotics, Control of—United States. I. Title
HV5825.S393   1992
363. 4'5'0973—dc20
                                                            92-53724
                                                                CIP

Dedicated to

S.C.

Contents

Acknowledgements

Of all the sections of the work, I think I approach this with this most trepidation, for fear a moment's lapse of memory will lead me to forget someone who labored a thankless hour, if not more, on this text. And for no better reason than that I asked them to.

Thanks to my enthusiastic and understanding committee chair, Tom Shibutani and John Baldwin, as well as Seth Fisher. I thank Sharon Collins and Constance McNeeley, who read early drafts of this work. I thank Bill Shay for starting me down this road, and Bob Niedeffer for his assistance and support. I would like to thank the many undergraduate students who offered their encouraging words.

I would like to thank David Watts for his thoughtful remarks. I would like to give a very special thanks to Julie Loehr of the Michigan State University Press, without whose priceless support this work could not have been.

Despite much help, no doubt errors remain. I am responsible for them all.

Preface

The specific purpose of this work is to analyze a social phenomenon, the "drug crisis." A string of words and phrases are typically used to characterize the problem; the "drug menace," "epidemic," "scourge," etc. Such words are so often repeated that their meaning has become unquestioned. The drug crisis is defined as a crisis of usage; of too many people making dangerous and illegal choices despite obvious health and public safety hazards. Why do people engage in such dangerous behavior? What could they be thinking of? How many must be arrested, politicians and the press wonder, before users get the message? So the storyline runs, a storyline relentlessly promoted by elected and appointed officials, and a storyline uncritically accepted and passed along by the media.

How can the "drug crisis" be understood, especially in all its aspects; the general perception of the crisis as well as the genuine substance of the crisis; the persistence of the users of illegal drugs; the frantic bidding war for greater expenditures against the "drug menace"; the various perspectives of dissent noted above and, equally, the imperviousness of public, press and politicians to professional criticism of the current policy? All of this put together is the "drug crisis." Is it possible to knit together one argument that can encompass the entirety of the crisis in its many substantive and symbolic aspects?

I believe so and the purpose of this work is to do just that. The critical argument is that illegal drug usage is very much rooted in legal drug usage. We are a society of members who routinely use drugs to maintain and enhance our lifestyle. In a sea of behavioral drug usage, a certain portion is contained and declared immoral and dangerous. Why should we be surprised that so many venture into the roped off area—particularly when drugs responsible for the deaths of one-half million Americans a year, alcohol and tobacco, are placed on the "safe" side of the line? Moreover, we are a society of members well-trained and well-encouraged in drug use. The line between legal and illegal is so often crossed precisely because taking a drug is perfectly compatible with standard American values and social practices.

This is made explicit in the opening chapter on the "medicine society." But this analysis is not enough. How is it that $15-20 billion annual law enforcement expenditures by Federal, state and local agencies has produced such meager results? How can drug marketeers defeat the combined forces of local, state and Federal police action? The "medicine society" explains the demand; it is still necessary to explain how it is that the supply side is flourishing despite the long and expensive "war against drugs."

In addition, the substantive and symbolic issues must be sorted through; what are the genuine facts and what are the spurious facts? How is it that the spurious facts have greater currency than the genuine facts? Why is it that 80 percent of users are white but 80 percent of defendants are people of color? After sorting through the genuine and the spurious, the substantive and the symbolic, what then is the real nature of the crisis? Further, why are Americans and their leaders so reluctant to peek behind the rhetoric and see what is real?

The need here is to synthesize research and commentary into one coherent argument against the status quo of current policy. A thoroughgoing social analysis is also called for. The drug crisis has deep roots. It is a particular society in a particular time and place that has produced this crisis—what is it about this society that produced and maintained the drug crisis? By "drug crisis" is meant the crisis in all its forms and diversions. It is not enough to solely analyze drug issues and policies; the society must be examined as well.

This might seem too large a task. Analysis of a society as large and dynamic as America's, however useful, even necessary it might appear to be, would seem beyond the scope of a work centering on the drug crisis. However, I would argue that the drug crisis itself can simplify and direct the task—the contemporary drug crisis can be the key that unlocks the nature of the society that produced the crisis. There must be a social analysis to fully understand the origins of the crisis—and the fact of the crisis itself can become the tool to illuminate the society. Further, the focus on the drug crisis simplifies the task of analysis—for we need only be concerned about those aspects of American society relevant to the task at hand.

The intent of this work, then, is to illuminate the crisis by making explicit the underlying conditions producing the crisis. Furthermore, the analysis intends to be useful—leading directly to policy recommendations that would mitigate the crisis. This leads to a third challenge—how can such an analysis plausibly be constructed?

Social analysis must of necessity face two challenges simultaneously; the analysis of the fact under study and then the analysis itself. How in the chaotic natural social universe is enough order found to justify the term "analysis"? The argument proceeds in the following way: first, factors generating the crisis will be proposed; second, the factors that should be mitigating, or diminishing, the crisis are examined. This examination will include the effects of drug laws and drug law enforcement as well as drug effects. Third, historical and cross-cultural data, as well as recent research findings, will be brought in as "real world" evidence of the facts and interacting effects of drug usage and drug policy. This is the broad outline of the analysis. The success of this approach is for the reader to decide.

There is one more critical point. Futurists tell us we live in a world in which the pace and scope of change is larger than ever before. the tools of knowledge, information, the computer, and the media have all combined to create this fact of change. Such change is presently chaotic, undirected and unplanned for. One outcome of such chaotic change is the drug crisis. But were we to choose to harness the tools of change and seek to deliberately direct the course of change—then we would empower ourselves to minimize, if not entirely eradicate, the crisis at hand. This, in brief, is the proposal embodied in this work.

Introduction

The bare facts of the drug crisis are these: in the final years of the 1980s, Americans spent approximately $50 billion a year on alcohol,[1] $40-50 billion on cocaine,[2] $35 billion a year for tobacco products,[3] $30 billion on prescription and over-the-counter drugs and preparations,[4] $25 billion a year on marijuana,[5] and $10-20 billion more on the rest of the illegal drugs.[6] In regard to the illegal drugs, these are conservative estimates. Yet even by a conservative estimate, Americans spent some $200 billion annually for their drugs. Of this, 85 percent was for legal and illegal behavioral drugs, drugs used solely to affect mood and to produce behavioral changes.

In comparison, 1988 annual personal expenditures were $500 billion for new housing, $450 billion for medical care, $250 billion for recreation and another $250 billion for clothes, $100 billion for new automobiles, and $100 billion for gasoline and oil. The combined drug industry is approximately equal to the auto and oil industry—and the drug industry in all its forms could well be larger. Drug sales are big business. The use of drugs, including illegal drugs, is as perfectly compatible with American values as the laws that would restrict or ban them.

This is not a new contradiction. What is different now is the cost of the contradiction; the cost in terms of underground market effects and the unintended consequences of enforcing the law. But even so, this is not the first time a prohibition proved of limited effectiveness. Using these figures, one way of visualizing current personal expenditures for drugs is to consider all of the new car dealerships in your community and then add in all gasoline and oil sales: the sales of legal and illegal behavioral drugs (alcohol, tobacco, sedative/hypnotics, and illicit drugs) will approximately equal the sales of the dealerships and outlets. Just as it is not the underclass supporting those auto dealerships, so too it is not the underclass that supports the legal and the illegal market in drugs. The underclass simply does not have the income to generate a market of that size.

In addition, consider the availability and sales of alcohol and cigarettes in your community; for alcohol, include sales from groceries, liquor stores, bars, and restaurants, and then include sales of all pharmaceuticals from local drug stores. Illegal drugs will do about the same dollar volume as those combined sales of cigarettes, alcohol, and pharmaceuticals, even though they are underground and out of sight. If anything, illegal drugs will have a greater sales volume. Furthermore, the illicit drugs are just about as available (for most people) as the legal behavioral drugs. Moreover, this is after a succession of political leaders have actively pressed a "war against drugs." Indeed, one of the peculiar and unintended consequences of this war and the way it has been waged is that for young people illicit drugs are probably more available than legal drugs.

What are the effects of such usage? In 1988, approximately 400,000 deaths were associated with tobacco usage, 100,000 deaths with alcohol usage, 5,000 deaths with prescription drug usage (primarily sedative/hypnotic or "sleeping pill" abuse)[7] and 3,500 deaths combined from all illegal drug usage (this, of course, includes heroin and "crack").[8] No deaths are associated with marijuana usage.

Of course, death rates are only one indicator of the number of individuals who suffer from the physical and psychological effects of drug usage. For example, in one study done at Johns Hopkins University, some 15-30 percent of all patients admitted to the hospital (some diagnosis other than drug or alcohol abuse) were found to be alcoholics. The difference in percentage depended upon the particular medical department into which the patients were admitted.[9] What is so often overlooked is that alcohol is not available because it is safe—it is widely available because Prohibition failed.

On one hand, it might make sense that legal drugs lead the list in lethality, simply due to availability. But the fact is, illegal drugs are virtually as available to most people. Secondly, while usage of illegal drugs has generated much hysteria, the lethality of tobacco, alcohol, and prescribed sedative/hypnotics has been virtually ignored by government officials responsible for the "war against drugs."

There has been a notable exception here—the work of former Surgeon General Everett Koop. Nonetheless, the tobacco industry remains a political power and even in a era where individuals, if not the government, deplore its usage, tobacco growers still command subsidies of hundreds of millions of dollars each year from the federal government.

Similarly, the alcohol industry remains a protected industry, with very little action taken to restrict the promotion of this drug. This is true even though much of its advertising appears to be targeted at young people, a population that cannot legally purchase the drug.

What are the trends? All usage rates are declining. Alcohol and tobacco were the first to show declines, tobacco beginning in 1977, alcohol in 1980. Marijuana followed, peaking in 1982. Cocaine usage began to fall in 1986. Overall, usage levels have dropped to the levels of 1973.

There are a number of caveats that must be added to this general picture. Only tobacco usage is in genuine decline, meaning its use is at a historical low. On the other hand, alcohol use has hardly declined, relative to its past usage rates. Furthermore, the use of illicit drugs, while in decline, nonetheless remains near historical peaks. Last, given stories of rising volumes of cocaine imports, the fact may be that people, given the current public climate, are less willing to report cocaine usage than in the past.

There are obvious exceptions to this general picture of declining usage. Even though general usage is declining, problematic usage, as measured by emergency room admissions due to drug overdoses, was on the increase until recently.[10] Regarding particulars, tobacco use is increasing among young women, generally but not exclusively among working-class women. Indeed, since 1986, deaths from lung cancer have exceeded deaths from breast cancer for American women.[11] In addition, there is a report that alcohol use is increasing among elementary school children; this age group is drinking at higher rates than previous generations and starting at a younger age. Generally though, the rise in problematic drug usage is limited to one group of people— the underclass.

These are the facts and contradictions of the "drug crisis." The purpose of this work is to explain or "diagnose" these facts and then propose solutions that would mitigate the crisis. There is the point of view that no such crisis exists. For example, in *The Nation*, the late Abbie Hoffman described the political posturing of the Reagan administration. Prior to the 1986 Congressional elections, the Reagan administration called for a "war against drugs." But after the election, they drafted a budget that cut one billion dollars from the "drug budget" and cut out all funds for drug treatment. Drug abuse is a genuine problem, Hoffman argued, but the "drug crisis" is no more than self-serving "hyperbole."[12]

Likewise, Adam Paul Weisman, in an article that appeared in *The New Republic*, "I was a Drug-Hype Junkie" (1986) wrote that the drug crisis "... was a perfect cover story: sensational, colorful, gruesome, alarmist, with a veneer of social responsibility. Unfortunately, it just wasn't true."[13] Weisman makes the argument that the usage of illegal drugs has been greatly sensationalized while the usage and harmful effects of legal drugs have been virtually ignored. He writes the real national problems are "...poverty, unemployment, illiteracy, malnutrition, murder and the Soviet Union."[14] These are the genuine issues, in this perspective, with the "drug crisis" a spurious issue, an issue that diverts rather than focuses attention.

Is there a genuine "crisis" or not? It is often said that the problem with economists is that they do not know the difference between good news and bad. By this it is meant that economists can explain why a rise in interest rates is good (even though it means loans are more expensive for everyone), and how a rise in the value of the dollar is bad (even though it means everyone's money is worth more than before). Nonetheless, most people know when there is an economic crisis, there are the simple measures of unemployment, inflation, and a rise in the Gross National Product; however murky the waters to a professional, to the public and political leaders, distinguishing good times from bad is pretty straightforward.

Social crises are another matter. We have lived so long with some crises—crime, poverty, and decaying cities—that we have stopped thinking of them as crises. They have become something else, acts of fate or God or the "invisible hand," beyond the ability of public action to remedy. Regarding the drug crisis, the murkiness includes: first, whether there is truly a "crisis," and second, the accuracy of the numbers that define the crisis. Then there is a third source of "murkiness": perhaps there is a "crisis" but of a quite different nature than usage per se. This opinion, the alternative to the standard opinion and to the opinions offered above, comes from Ethan Nadelmann, perhaps the leading proponent of this view.

Nadelmann argues that there is a genuine drug crisis, but that it resides in the underground market effects of official corruption and in the law enforcement effects of overloading the criminal justice system. This is the genuine crisis, he argues, rather than the consequences of the usage of drugs far less lethal than the official drugs of choice. His clear statement of the problem has made his writing the critical voice for this position.

Further, all of these points of view express concern over the constriction of individual liberty. We live in a time when ordinary and traditional sorts of freedom, such as freedom from unreasonable searches and seizures, are being reduced to enhance police action. Indeed, Milton Friedman, conservative economist and Nobel Prize winner, states the reductions in individual liberties being performed in the name of greater police efficiency vis-a-vis the drug crisis is the genuine "crisis," rather than drug usage per se.[15]

The question is not which opinion is right or wrong: social life is too ambiguous to fit into that frame. The better question is what opinion is most useful to mitigating the "crisis"? By "drug crisis" it is meant the crisis in all its forms, including drug usage and the effect of the drug laws. The question must also be: what opinion is most consistent with the best of American traditions and values? Then the question becomes: how is the opinion to be hammered into the form of public policy?

However murky economics might be, how much more so is the study of a society. An economy can be measured in discrete dollars, rendering its facts (if not the interpretations) to consensus. Social behavior, on the other hand, finds a poor reflection in numbers. Moreover, the person passing judgement based upon the numbers must always remember that these numbers are responses to a survey asking individuals to honestly report their not respectable and even illegal behavior. These numbers are then interpreted by administrators whose career paths will be determined by program growth. The numbers themselves are suspect and this redoubles the potential for controversy.

A clear argument, an argument that addresses two sorts of issues simultaneously, is needed. One sort of issue is the substantive: here, a straightforward and traditional approach is offered, mitigating the social ill by effecting change in the society that nourished the crisis. A second set of issues deals with the frame of the argument itself—how does one go about creating such an argument? How is public policy sensibly constructed from the unsteady materials of flawed data and biased judgement, including the bias of the critic?

There is some steady ground here. There are the current facts measured against the past. There is a history to consult, both in this country and overseas. Where are we, not only in terms of the "crisis," but equally in terms of the larger issues of social change that can plausibly be relevant to the crisis?

What has worked in the past and what has not? What has worked for other countries with a similar crisis? How, in the opinion of experts from a number of relevant disciplines and professions, is present policy working and not working? Though each and every block of opinion and research that might be brought to bear comes with a certain degree of ambiguity and bias, nonetheless, a certain consensus can be discerned, a consensus consistent with past history and present facts. These are the basic building blocks of the argument presented here.

The author accepts here that the drug crisis is genuine. This crisis exists within a particular society; a society with a profound belief in the efficacy of "drugs" and a long history of tolerance to mainstream drug usage. This is a society of members who routinely use "drugs" of whatever sort to maintain and enhance their individual lifestyle, who use alcohol/drugs as social lubricants and as the center of their celebrations, both large and small. This is the medicine society. Given such a society, we would expect to find a drug crisis and we do.

But there is not only a drug crisis, there is more going on than that. Most individuals exercise individual sensibility and judgement and limit their use. This judgement, exercised individually and collectively, is the "natural healer." "Natural healer" means that even as penicillin does not "cure" infection so much as it aids the body's own immunosystem, and even as a cast does not "heal" a broken bone so much as help the body to heal itself, so too public policy must be about aiding the natural defense of individual decision-making. Moreover, without the natural healer of individual sensibility there would be no need to talk of social crisis, but only because there would hardly be this thing called society.

In regards to the drug crisis, how can a public policy be constructed to aid the "natural healer" of individual sensibility? This leads to a second question: How can public policy be constructed to mitigate the effects of individuals who do not (on occasion or persistently) exercise sound and sensible judgement?

Modern societies have institutionalized responses to such ills as the drug crisis—a public health system. Such an institution would mitigate emerging health problems by early detection and by deploying a pre-existing system of hospitals, clinics and treatment staffs of whatever kind. In this way, a crisis is contained, headed off before the problem can become a crisis. Moreover, funding is provided the helping professions for public education and information, the goal being to prevent such problems from occurring. This might sound all too obvious and commonsensical to be worth stating, but the fact is the United States does not have such a system.

Rather, hospitals in underclass neighborhoods are closing their doors (this is so even as their beds are full), and mental health clinics and drug treatment centers are being shut down, not expanded, because of a lack of funding. Even emergency rooms, those critical health care providers, are besieged by red ink because of the health care costs of providing for the uninsured and are suffering the same fate as hospitals and clinics.

Rather than being empowered to mitigate the drug crisis, the public health system is itself in crisis. Nor is the drug crisis the only facet of the larger crisis. Infant mortality rates are at Third World rates in many of the underclass neighborhoods of America. If only white infants' rates were considered, these would still rank near the bottom of the developed world's mortality rates. Further, malnutrition, an evil eliminated in much of the underdeveloped world, is a critical problem in the United States.[16] Moreover, this was a social ill we had once nearly eliminated. There are many such crises but there is really only one crisis with many faces—the crisis in public health.

Present policy is the police and preacher option. Americans have a childlike faith in the efficacy of preaching to the individual. This is the traditional American approach to the challenge of social crisis and change. In this way, the challenge of dealing with changing times can be evaded and deflected to the police station and the pulpit. But police action, a social policy by default, can only suppress the worst of the symptoms while generating yet new ones as court dockets and prisons fill with the usual suspects; the poor, the uneducated and the Americans of color. Hence the crisis goes on, undermining both the social health and the social peace.

There have been alternatives. At the turn of the century, clinics were the prime social response to the treatment of addiction. The government, curiously, actively worked to shut down the clinics. This is a history worth noting. In 1914 the Harrison Act was passed. Previously, narcotics had been openly sold over-the-counter or through the mail. After 1914 they could be legally possessed only via a prescription. The newly formed Narcotics Bureau was displeased with this and pressed the Supreme Court to outlaw heroin maintenance, the accepted medical practice of the time for the treatment of addiction. The Court was to comply in a series of decisions, a history David Musto details in The American Disease (1987).[17]

At the time, a number of treatment clinics for narcotics addiction were operating in the United States. But the physicians directing the clinics were under constant pressure from the Bureau to shut their doors and most did, however reluctantly. Yet some held out.

One target of the Narcotics Bureau in 1919 was the Shreveport Clinic, operated by a Dr. Butler. The initial report from the Narcotics Bureau field agents praised the clinic and its founder. There was not a single prescription found in local drugstores for addicts. Instead, local druggists, physicians, elected officials, the police chief, and the Federal District Judge of the region all praised the clinic. Indeed, the unanimous opinion was that "...they were no longer bothered by drug addicts except an occasional visitor to the city."[18] The local police were concerned that if the clinic was closed, the problem of an underground market would begin to surface.

The Bureau was not impressed (though its own field agents were) and this clinic, one of the last resisters, was closed. This is the history of an obscure Washington-based law enforcement bureau determining proper medical practice in opposition to the opinion of physicians. Of course, the use of Federal power to determine medical practices, even when contrary to the best medical advice, continues today; referring to a recent law that forbids open dialogue between physician and patient when the issue is pregnancy and abortion.

There is one other variable, the vacuum of leadership on the part of the White House and Congress, a vacuum created by elected officials who hesitate to factually and responsibly address a controversial issue. Moreover, even as this is history, it is also current. The circumstances today have not changed a bit. This is why we are undergoing yet another "drug crisis."

Briefly, what is the analysis and the proposals to be presented here? The lack of public health is the "Achilles' heel" of social peace. It is public health that mitigates poverty, provides an alternative crime control and, by nurturing the future generation, helps preserve the individual initiative that makes real political and economic opportunity possible. When public health is in crisis, none of these functions are fulfilled.

It is not that public health can reverse these social ills, but it is public health that can make a difference in individuals making a difference in their own lives. Public health mitigates; lacking this mitigation, there can be no chance of social peace.

A meager commitment to public health has become the American norm. This was not always the case. Indeed, the notion and practice of modern public health was invented in this country. Furthermore, it is no accident that as we have abandoned public health, our poverty and crime rates have become the highest in the developed world.

After World War II, every Western European country established a comprehensive health care program for their citizens. Indeed, the difference was only one of degree over the system already present. This was one of the effects of the War: a democratization of health care. Yet in the United States, health care remained the domain of private health plans. Today, 17 percent of the American population has no health plan, meaning this many are doing without any health care at all.

How do Americans explain their poverty and crime rate? There is a traditional American response here as well: such rates are the fault of the minority population. This is what minorities are good for—scapegoats for problems we all do our fair share to create. Present-day minorities should not take it personally; in the 1920s, when the minorities were the Irish, the Italian, and the Jewish people, they too were made good use of. It is only a short step to use the same people as scapegoats for the drug problems of an era and then claim one problem, drugs, creates the other of crime. Hence, in the coverage of the "drug crisis," faces and neighborhoods of the underclass are featured, despite the classless and raceless nature of the problem. The drug crisis is a crisis we all, or most of us, have done our fair share to create.[19]

We are fortunate to have the minority teenager on the streetcorner to point out as the scapegoat of this crisis. But blaming this stereotype, however good it feels, has yet to resolve the crisis. The difficulty is that the scenario is half-right. There is a drug crisis in the underclass (and here "underclass" is used in its most general meaning, the poor). But the difference between the underclass and those covered by health plans is not to be found in excessive drug use for that is found in every sort of place and person. Instead the difference is that young people growing up in underclass neighborhoods have no access to effective health care. The difference is one of the availability of relief; the generator of the problem works across class.

This does not absolve the young people of the underclass (or any people) from individual responsibility. The point is that individual responsibility is expressed by seeking help and therapy when one recognizes one has a problem. However, in the underclass neighborhood, the person who exercises individual initative and seeks help will find little, for health care professionals are scarce resources in these neighborhoods.

There is one critical reason for that. Such care is paid for through private health plans. Those who stand outside such plans are denied a genuine benefit of participation in the American system, that of having access to the most advanced medicine and medical care in the world. Those who stand outside of such a benefit stand outside of such a system. Public health is as precious as the vote.

Public health is the mitigator; the generator of the "drug crisis" can be found in everyday American social practices and beliefs. It is perfectly compatible in this culture for members to take a drug. If the weakness of American society is a lack of public health, a strength is the production of "miracle drugs." Post-World War II, generation after generation of Americans have benefitted from continual pharmaceutical invention. Drugs work, drug usage produces cures, this is why the belief in the efficacy of drugs is so difficult to overturn. It is generally founded on solid fact.

Moreover, this culture does not stop there. Madison Avenue, the social psychologist of the public mind, is an apt persuader of the virtues of behavioral drugs, particularly alcohol. Madison Avenue sells alcohol by attempting to persuade individuals that the use of alcohol can solve their personal and social problems. If one needs friends, if one wishes to have a "good time," use alcohol. This is the constant message of television advertisement, including (especially) those on professional sports programs, a favorite of young people.

It is not possible for science to verify the harmful effects of such persuasion; consider that science will not even verify that cigarette use produces lung cancer, nor that taking aspirin "causes" a lowering of body temperature. The standard of proof and cause used in positive science is too high to be matched by any sort of research into behavior. But we can trust that business people are knowledgeable in what they do and would not spend billions of dollars in advertisements if such expenditures did not work.

Beginning in the first chapter of Part One, the aspects of the medicine society will be presented as generating the crisis. In addition, there has been in our time an internationalization of travel, trade and preferences: the market internationale. The underground market does not stand apart from that internationalization, rather, like all trade, the underground market is prospering within internationalization. Further, futurists and social commentators inform us that this internationalized society is undergoing profound change of another sort, an evolution (many would say revolution) of the post-modern. This too, along with the failure to recognize and respond to such changes, plays a role in generating the drug crisis.

In Part Two, the public health crisis and the contradictions of the public policy of law enforcement are offered as reasons for the failure of alleviating the crisis. In addition, this question must be addressed—what are the problems associated with drug usage? Does the problem warrant the given cure? The literature on drug usage will be reviewed, focusing upon the behavioral effects of drug usage and reports upon the link between usage and crime. The literature on the effectiveness of drug treatment and education will also be reviewed.

Part Three examines the effects on the underground market and law enforcement effects created by the current policy. As this is not the first drug crisis in American history, nor is America the only country with a drug problem, past crises in U.S. history and present drug crises in comparable countries will be examined. The aim here is to find out the successful solutions and the failed attempts. In other words, we should know what has worked and what has not worked. In the last chapter, the argument will be summed up, with public policy recommendations included in the summary.

The final question relevant to this introduction must be: What of the problem of personal bias? Supposedly, the facts are selected on the subject, placed in logical order and this results, it is said, in the facts speaking for themselves without the intervention of subjective prejudice. But this is the ideal. Few claim such a description matches the actual doing of any project, including the projects of science. What is dismissed as only prejudice equally contains the critical factor of judgement, without which no determination can be made.

Nonetheless, the problem of bias remains. The author does not claim to be without it. No doubt the argument was generally conceived before the serious collection of facts began. Those facts, rather than helping to build the argument, filled in the gaps or made more explicit just what the argument was always going to be. So the aim is not to claim innocence, but rather to make the argument worth your attention, even given the presence of unintended bias.

Moreover, as will be seen, part of this bias is to maintain that this is the era of change, when change itself, of whatever kind and in whatever direction, is more possible than it has ever been. This is a distilled opinion of what "post-modern" or "post-industrial" means to public policy. This is encouraging. Even as social change and unintended consequences have generated the drug crisis, there is equally the potential for a proactive public policy to mitigate the social ill and provide for the social peace. The intent of this work is to participate in that discourse.

Notes

1. Weldon Witters and Peter Venturelli, *Drugs and Society* (Boston: Jones and Bartlett, 1988), 12.
2. Peter Reuter, Gordon Crawford and Jonathan Cave, *Sealing the Borders*, R-3594-USDP (Santa Monica: RAND National Defense Research Institute, 1988). Reuter estimated $25 billion personal expenditures for cocaine in 1985. The $50 billion figure used here is based on Reuter's estimate for 1985, plus the later increase in estimates of the volume of imported cocaine, plus considering the decline in the wholesale price of cocaine and then adjusting for inflation.
3. U.S. Bureau of the Census, *Statistical Abstract of the U.S. 1989,* No. 693 (Washington, DC: U.S. Government Printing Office, 1989), 426.
4. Ibid.
5. Witters and Venturelli, *Drugs and Society,* 13.
6. Ibid.
7. Ibid., 181.
8. Ibid., 233.
9. Richard D. Moore, et al., "Prevention, Detection and Treatment of Alcoholism in Hospitalized Patients," *Journal of the American Medical Association* 261(20 January 1989): 403-8.
10. "Cocaine Related Deaths Decline for First Time in a Decade, Federal Figures Reveal," *Los Angeles Times,* 21 May 1990. The report was

based upon National Institute of Drug Abuse (NIDA) data.

11. "Under Fire: Women and Smoking," *Los Angeles Times,* 17 April 1990.

12. Abbie Hoffman, "Reefer Madness," *The Nation,* 21 November 1987, 580.

13. Adam Paul Weismann, "I was a Drug-Hype Junkie," *The New Republic,* 6 October 1986, 15.

14. Ibid.

15. Milton Friedman, "An Open Letter to Bill Bennett," *Wall Street Journal,* 7 September 1989.

16. Larry J. Brown, "Hunger in the U.S.," *Scientific American* 256 (February 1987): 37-41. See also Timothy M. Smeeding and Barbara Boyld Torrey, "Poor Children in Rich Countries," *Science* 243 (November 1988): 873-77.

17. David Musto, *The American Disease,* 2nd ed. (New Haven: Yale University Press, 1987). Regarding the Harrison Act, see also Alfred Lindesmith, *The Addict and the Law* (Bloomington: Indiana University Press, 1965); Troy Duster, The Legislation of Morality (New York: Free Press, 1970).

18. David Musto, *The American Disease,* 2nd ed. (New Haven: Yale University Press, 1987), 168.

19. Besides David Musto's standard work, see also William Foote Whyte's, *Street Corner Society* (Chicago: University of Chicago Press, 1943) for a description of an Italian community that exactly parallels today's conventional description of the "inner-city" neighborhood.

Part One

Factors Generating the "Drug Crisis"

1

The Medicine Society

In the waters of the Caribbean, there is a fish of the genus *Spheroides*, otherwise called the pufferfish. This fish produces a toxin that has the following unusual effect in humans: a temporary but total paralysis virtually indistinguishable from death, a paralysis made more remarkable by the fact that the victims remains totally conscious during their ordeals.

Such an effect is too tempting for social beings such as ourselves to let alone. The Haitians (it is conjectured) use this drug as an agent of social control and punishment: deviants are punished by having this drug administered surreptitiously and, are thereby, turned into "zombies." Presumably, this inoculation of socialization produces satisfactory results in both the disturbers and the champions of the social peace. This is not the only use of the pufferfish. The Japanese, who seem, at times, to be connoisseurs of anything remotely dangerous, like to eat the fish raw. That the preparation is not always successful is how we know the fish causes such paralysis.

For the purposes of this work, what is critical is this example of a physiological effect that is used as a resource by members of a society and transformed into a sociological effect. Hence, a drug effect is turned into social meaning and woven into the fabric of everyday life as well as into the larger social and political context of everyday life.

Our use of drugs is no different. The drug usage of American society cannot be understood simply in terms of pharmacological substances and physiological effects; rather, such usage must be understood in the context of our everyday and our larger social and political life. To divorce drug use from that context is to entirely misunderstand usage. Even the assumption that there is a specific physiological effect that produces, in turn, a definitive effect called a "high" is suspect. What is a "high"? We can find evidence of unusual alpha wave activity, but the truth is we can neither define nor demonstrate a "high," however much we are certain to know it when we feel it.

The best we can do is to go out and ask people what they think it is and how it feels. But such research simply restates what our own subjectivity tells us, or we end up with results that report back outdated research that has seeped into popular discourse. In either case, we are left no more knowledgeable than when we started.

Socially defined effects are particularly true of alcohol. By particularly, it is meant that this drug in particular is woven into the social fabric simply by virtue of its longer and more extensive history relative to other mood and behavioral drugs. Given that history, it is also the most reported upon of drugs. Certain physiological effects such as vasodilation, the metabolism of alcohol to acetaldehyde, can be documented and shown as universally true with whatever variations (for example, the metabolization of alcohol occurs somewhat differently in individuals of Asian ancestry). But in regard to a property such as impaired judgement or disinhibition, both commonly attributed to alcohol, it is much less clear that this is a straightforward physiological effect.

This issue was the subject of a conference held at Berkeley in 1981. The conclusion, consistent with findings from a number of different fields, was "...to suggest that the link between alcohol and disinhibition is a matter of *cultural belief* rather than of *pharmacological action*" [emphasis author's].[1] We certainly feel different after a drink but "how we interpret those feelings, and in particular how we act upon them, is largely determined by culture and circumstance."[2]

Moreover, in our particular culture, regardless of particular circumstances, when people drink alcohol they then use alcohol to explain their own and other's behavior. This use of alcohol is a social product and not simply the outcome of a physiological process.[3] Nor does the mystique surrounding alcohol stop there. Barbara Critchlow Leigh points out: "Alcohol is expected to result in increased relaxation, power, sociability, behavioral impairment and sexual enhancement; in general, people believe that alcohol changes them in many ways."[4] All of these effects are relevant to socializing. Alcohol helps people "do" social relationships, or so they believe, which is, in effect, one and the same thing.

Moreover, Leigh's report is typical of those in the field; there is a rather large consensus on this point. For example, Frieze and Schafer make the point that the physiological effects of alcohol, such as vasodilation and increased heart rate, tend to be "...interpreted as feelings of emotional warmth by a woman and as feelings of power by a man given sex-role socialization."[5]

The now familiar theme here is that physiological effects become translated into psychological and sociological effects. And it is these effects that become central to the experiencing and meaning of the drug. In other words, the physiological effects are trivial, save that they are used as a basis to produce the social effects.[6] Of course, the social-psychological effects are no illusion: the social effects are as real as any physiological effects. Given the effects reported, combined with the fact that any social improprieties or mishaps are going to be excused if performed after the consumption of alcohol, and then given that both parties involved (the doer and the observer or receiver of the impropriety) share the same attitude, this amounts to a license to either be improper or to at least be unconcerned and without the usual anxiety over the social costs and sanctions of acting out-of-line. Hence, alcohol's positive effect on sociability becomes a social fact and an equally valuable resource to the "doing" of social relationships.

Individuals often experience alcohol (as well as any number of drugs, particularly cocaine and marijuana) as aphrodiasical. This is experienced as a physiological effect but, once again, researchers discredit this. Alan R. Lang reports "...to the extent drugs function as aphrodiasiacs, this effect is often more a psychosocial 'remission' or 'excuse' to feel and act sexual than a direct pharmacological stimulation or disinhibition of physiological sexual response."[7]

He further notes that in experimental studies "...the belief that one is intoxicated has been shown to increase physiological and subjective sexual arousal in men, while women's reports of sexual pleasure often correspond to their level of intoxication."[8] Lang goes on to report that the physiological evidence of alcohol being an aphrodisiac is "embarrassed by the evidence."[9]

Sexual and social revolutions come and go, but American squeamishness regarding sexuality and a fundamentally Victorian suspicion of sexuality endures. American society is one whose members may well need the social-psychological effects of alcohol and drug ingestion to enjoy their sexuality or, at least, many members act as if this were the case. Those social-psychological effects are the aphrodiasical effects; they are genuine in that they are experienced as genuine, with the physiological facts of the matter being of little relevance. Further, given that drinking is accompanied by a relaxation of the usual everyday norms and conventions, we can appreciate that drinking, if not the alcohol itself, is, however paradoxically, a genuine aphrodisiac even if not by any physiological measure.

Is there a generalization we can draw from the research? This one is offered: impaired judgement and disinhibition is believed by individuals to be a physiological effect, beyond an individual's volition or deliberate doing, and this belief in turn is used by us as a critical foundation in our socializing. Hence (following Barbara Leigh primarily): the crucial social fact of drinking is that we are relieved of responsibility for our behavior by others; we relieve ourselves of responsibility, and at the same time, we relieve others of their individual responsibility for behavior. In a real sense, this could be why we are having a drink and how we come to equate having a "party" with drinking. Further, this can be understood as critical to our sexual expression, to our giving ourselves permission to enjoy our sexuality.

Socially then, a drink is magic. Having a drink in one's hand effects a magical transformation of status from being a person who is held accountable for his or her behavior to being a person who is free from any such constraints, who grants such freedom to others and equally expects to be granted that license by others.

We stand ready to excuse almost any behavior by ourselves or others so long as it was performed under the influence of a drink. Furthermore, we all understand that this excuse will be given for us and we stand ready to use this social fact as a reason for doing what we might otherwise stop ourselves from doing. Being expert and adept members of society, does it not make sense that we would freely make use of this social artifact, a drink, and thereby transport ourselves into a freer and more gratifying (at least temporarily) social sphere?

A further point is that drug usage is not on the periphery of our personal and social life. For most of us, drug usage is at the very center of our socializing, and of our social celebrations both large and small. When a group of friends gets together in shared companionship, a drug is produced (legal or not), as a token of the circumstance of shared informal friendship. Sharing in the euphoric and social effects of drugs, or effects experienced as such, is how people drop the mirrors and masks of the everyday, the conventional and the structured, and relate as more "genuine" and more "open" individuals. To do so is, in fact, the very reason they use the drug. Of course, such facts are not just true of alcohol. These sorts of expectations, beliefs, motives, and experiences, are social-psychological and quite immune to any legal ramifications.

This is critical to understanding the origin of the "drug crisis." In a sea of behavioral drug use, a certain segment is roped off and declared dangerous, immoral, and criminal. But legal usage does not exist in a vacuum. Rather, such usage is constructed and maintained by any number of enduring social beliefs and practices, each one of which is equally capable of justifying the usage of illegal drugs. Indeed, all the myths and uses of alcohol as relaxant, disinhibitor, aphrodisiac, as well as the social signifier of being informal, in celebration, outside everyday conventions, all the pre-existing social facts that are actively promoted and maintained by Madison Avenue, all can and do get applied to other drugs as well. Why should anyone be surprised at how new drugs are continually added to the crisis—we are a society of members who have been well-prepared and well-trained in the social uses of drugs.

Nor is the medicine society limited to mood and behavioral drugs. Another facet of the drug problem is the use by young people of anabolic steroids to enhance the cosmetics of body shape and muscle definition as well as to gain strength and improve performance. In the first national survey of steroid use (46 high schools, 3,403 students surveyed), 6.6 percent of high school seniors reported using such drugs. Two-thirds had used steroids by the age of 16 or before, 40 percent of users reported using the drug for at least five cycles (each cycle is 6 to 12 weeks long). Most took the drug to improve athletic performance, 27 percent took the drug solely to enhance personal appearance.[10]

The authors of this American Medical Association article extrapolated a figure of 500,000 young people who have used anabolic steroids. Since this is the most extensive survey ever done, it is the most precise data available. In the literature there are higher estimates, the highest figure given being 1 million users annually, with 5 percent of college athletes and 7 to 8 percent of professional athletes reported as users.[11]

There are also reports of users becoming psychologically dependent upon the drug, perhaps more accurately put as dependent on the taking of the drug.[12] The physiological and behavioral effects of the drug cannot readily account for dependency but, evidently, the act of taking the drug becomes a learned response best explained by classical conditioning; the drug-taking, by itself, comes to be equated by the user with enhanced appearance and athletic performance. A caveat should be added here: the drug does have mood and behavioral effects, for example increased aggressiveness, and as people can become dependent upon the relaxant effects of any number of drugs, perhaps people can also become dependent upon an aggressive effect. In any case, drug usage is never simply physiological.

Even as the drug crisis is not limited to mood and behavioral drugs, so too the underlying social psychology of usage extends beyond such effects. We equate drugs with cure and, again, this is no illusion. We believe drugs work because drugs do work. Since World War II, we have benefitted from an apparently unceasing output of new and efficacious "miracle" drugs. Infections, diseases, pain, all have been relieved and many diseases entirely eradicated by the introduction of a new drug. Drugs work, people equate drugs with cure and when they visit their physician are often not relieved until and unless they leave the office with a prescription. Now, in many cases, there could well be better alternatives to particular health problems, such as a change in diet or an increase in exercise, but, generally, the patient wants a pill and the doctor is happy to oblige. This person who is the patient is, of course, us.

We do not only look to drugs to cure as individuals; at the social level, whenever a medical problem emerges, be it Acquired Immune Deficiency Syndrome (AIDS) or even the problem of drug addiction, the cry repeated in newspapers and journals is for the "magic bullet" that will cure the problem. And this is, again, entirely sensible, for recent history is full of the success stories of such "magic bullets."

Indeed, those diseases that remain beyond the reach of cure, such as cancers, are precisely those diseases that have proved to be beyond the reach of any such "magic bullet." It is maintained here that the belief that drugs cure is yet another example of a type of thinking, an underlying social belief and practice that is the infrastructure of the medicine society. This is an infrastructure that accommodates the usage of illegal drugs as readily as the usage of legal drugs. We are a society of members who do not fear drugs; on the contrary, drugs are equated with positive effects and positive outcomes.

In point of fact, we routinely use drugs to maintain and enhance our lifestyle. This is true of mood and behavioral drugs (whether legal or illegal) but also generally true of all drug use. The best example is the birth control pill. Whether the introduction of birth control pills triggered the sexual revolution of the 1960s and 1970s, or indeed whether there really was such a revolution, is not unanimously agreed upon. Reasonable people can agree that there was a change, a change toward greater sexual activity, and a change that was sparked in part by birth control pills. Whether this change amounted to a revolution can be safely left to historians, sociologists, and psychologists (not to resolve but to happily argue).

Nonetheless, here is pharmaceutical technology altering culture and doing so because a drug such as birth control pills, in their social aspect, is located in the most sensitive areas of individuality and culture: our health, sexuality, and social relationships. Though adverse risks have been extensively publicized (and, of course, debated by medical scientists, such as the real increased risk of ovarian cancer following years of birth control pill usage), still, in 1985, 50 million prescriptions were filled (down from 60 million in 1982) and used by approximately 15 million women (down from 25 million in 1973). Of those women who stopped using birth control pills (or never used them), other medical options such as sterilization or other sorts of contraceptives were chosen. Precious few of us, whether male or female, choose to close the doors opened by the sexual revolution (that is, if those doors were ever as closed as cultural memory might have us believe).

Drugs are a critical technology, often overlooked when technology is understood to mean computers, communications, or hardware of whatever sort. Drugs can be considered part of our cultural software, an "invisible hand" shaping our choices and social practices in immediate and profound ways. We have grown accustomed to this drug usage and find little remarkable in it.

Birth control pills are a good example of another aspect of the "drug crisis": the lack of good health information. What are the health consequences, for example, of birth control pill usage? Here science's standards of proof are more of a hindrance than a help. Why is it so difficult for medical science to offer women sound advice? According to the same research referenced, regarding women who quit the pill: "Explicit medical advice played a less critical role in pill discontinuation than did women's independent judgement. Just over one-third of former users had been told by a doctor to stop using the pill."[13]

Women, with their intense networks, networks that extend into mass culture and produce innumerable women's magazines, get around the lack of good information by turning to themselves. It is questionable whether doctors or medical science is to blame for the lack of clear information. What is of relevance here is that the lack of sound information and the lack of a means of communicating that information is typical of this country, given the lack of a public health system. This lack extends into behavioral drug usage, whether legal or illegal.

Anti-drug campaigns tout education, not that this produces more funding for it. What is overlooked is that the lack of useful health information is typical of the American way of public health. Without a public health authority intent upon getting usable information into people's hands (such as former Surgeon General Everett Koop's anti-smoking campaign), public ignorance must be corrected by private resources and initiative, with all the uncertainty, inconsistency, and bias (meaning that the poor are often left out of the information loop) that is to be expected and is perfectly consistent with the general lack of American public health.

Birth control is useful for illuminating other aspects of the drug crisis. Birth control devices (including pills) were illegal to sell in a number of states; it was even illegal to provide birth control information. This did not change until the rather late date of 1965, in the Supreme Court decision *Griswold v. Connecticut*. In this case, two officers of a planned parenthood league were arrested and fined in Connecticut for giving out birth control information to a married couple. The Court overturned the conviction, invoking a "right to privacy," or using Justice Brandeis' (1890) term (as the Court did), "the right to be left alone." This right became the basis of *Roe v. Wade*, the 1973 landmark abortion ruling.[14]

To continue this story just a bit: Planned Parenthood was founded by Margaret Sanger in 1914-15. Her first article on such was banned in the United States and she was arrested for "misuse of the mail." The charges were dropped. However, when she and her sister opened their first clinic, the clinic was closed by the police and both were arrested and convicted for "maintaining a public nuisance." The appeals court overturned the verdict and ruled that doctors could give out such information but providing it was only for the purpose of disease prevention.

This particular story was about birth control devices rather than drugs, but the story has a certain relevance to the drug crisis. There are two complementary points here, beyond what has already been noted about the medicine society. First, what might be regarded as a straightforward matter of public health is instead regarded as a moral issue. This was true of birth control, was true of AIDS, and is also true of the drug crisis. Second, individuals may seek to rectify social ills via social activism, but when they do so they are quite likely to find a government that actively prohibits their work.

The American public and their politicians insist upon a moral definition of these issues and this definition disinhibits health funding and effective remedies. At the social level, such thinking is self-defeating. Prohibition failed to solve the problem of alcoholism, moralizing about homosexuality failed to halt AIDS, and moralizing about birth control usage only intruded upon a fundamental understanding of Americans' relationships to their government, the "right to be left alone." Moralisms regarding the drug crisis are similarly unhelpful. For evidence, one need only note that there has been considerable moralizing, yet the crisis remains. How can moralizing work to mitigate the drug crisis when there is a fundamental hypocrisy to all such moralizing?

Drug use is pervasive, but only a particular type of use is separated from general usage and labeled as a moral usage. For example, no moral frame is applied to sedative/hypnotics. Being legal, in the public mind, is evidently equated with being safe and being moral. In the 1986 ABC Drug Abuse Poll (based upon a phone survey of 2,326 individuals),[15] more people had used sedatives/hypnotics than any illegal behavioral drug. Furthermore, when asked about the dangers of the behavioral drugs they used, sedative/hypnotics were thought to be less dangerous than, for example, marijuana and cocaine.

In fact, one type of sedative/hypnotic, barbiturates, "...are probably involved in three-fourths of all deaths (accidental or suicide) for drugs, currently estimated at 5,000 deaths per year"[16] (here the authors are referring to legal prescription drug usage). Yet no moral frame is applied to such usage. For comparison, the annual toll of all illegal drug usage combined is estimated to be 3,500 deaths, less than sedative/hypnotics. The same point, of course, could be made for cigarettes and alcohol.

The point here is not that the illegal drugs, most commonly marijuana or cocaine, are "safe." Marijuana is a relatively innocuous

drug, particularly compared to cocaine or alcohol, but it is not a
health drug; the inhalation of smoke alone is damaging to health.
Further, any drug that induces desirable behavioral effects (attributed to physiology but again, social psychology is more often the
genuine effect), brings with it the problem of dependency.

The point regarding sedative/hypnotics is this: when individuals
use a sedative/hypnotic, they are using a drug that is more dangerous (by mortality statistics and dependency statistics) than marijuana, yet there are neither legal nor moral stigmas attached to
such usage. Such hypocrisy is as much a part of the medicine society as drug usage itself. This hypocrisy in turn helps drive the crisis as current laws and regulations, being so contrary to
experience and fact, are much more easily ignored.

Regarding Sanger's struggle to establish planned parenthood
clinics and, closer to our time, the illegalization of birth control
information and devices, there is a second parallel that can be
drawn to the drug crisis: individuals may seek to cure social ills
through individual action but they often will not find a helpful, or
even neutral, government. Indeed, they may find a government
that actively prohibits their work. Such was the case in the government's response to the first drug treatment clinics established
in the country—the drug enforcement agency of the era shut them
down. The Shreveport clinic story was noted in the introduction
but Shreveport was only the last to close. Many cities had drug
treatment clinics; all were forced to close in the years 1919-21.[17]

These clinics were for heroin addicts primarily. The clinics
were closed because the Narcotics Division objected to the then
standard method of treating heroin—providing addicts with
heroin in steadily decreasing doses. In addition, such treatment,
when not successful, provided for continuing the addict on
clinic-supplied doses. The reasoning, as noted in the introduction, was that failure to treat addicts would create yet more problems, primarily the commission of crimes by addicts to obtain
money for their supply and the creation of an underground market with all the additional crime such markets support. Even
when the public and local officials supported the clinics, they
were closed by the Bureau.

The relevance of this story is: we cannot simply leave the story
at the point of generalized social beliefs and practices impersonally
shaping public policy. Rather, we find specific bureaucracies,
such as the Narcotics Bureau, the earlier version of the current
Drug Enforcement Agency (DEA), actively seeking to expand their

turf. Given the power of any bureaucracy of the Federal government, when the Federal agency collides with professional and
local opinion, it is the latter that gives. Hence, we have an example of an obscure Washington bureaucracy successfully expanding
into the medical treatment of drug addiction over the objections of
both the medical profession and local officials, including police
and judges. The present story with the DEA is no different.

Nonetheless, however gratifying it is to point the finger at a particular government agency and place the blame there, the crisis is
too severe and widespread to leave the argument there. First,
whatever the proposed solutions to the drug crisis, law enforcement has a role to play, few propose a complete abolition of regulation. Second, part of the blame must lie with the law and the
policymakers that direct law enforcement.

Certainly such agencies as the DEA, as is true of any bureaucracy, are prone to turf jealousy and seek to expand their administrative areas at the expense of other agencies and concerns.
Nonetheless, this does not mean that public officials are duty-
bound to passively accept such expansion. Drug education and
drug treatment clinics could just as easily be expanded as law
enforcement. Yet a vacuum of executive and congressional leadership is typical in this drug crisis and, moreover, typical of the previous drug crises of Victorian and pre-World War II America. Nor
does the blame stop there. The question becomes, how are the contradictory laws and attitudes—the contradictions that ultimately
undermine law enforcement and will continue to do so no matter
how much money is spent—to be resolved? Furthermore, how is
the passivity of law and policymakers to be accounted for?

The consensus of researchers who have studied the question is
that the differences of legal status among many substances is
social, not physiological or pharmacological. One sort of substance
is used by the middle-class and the well-to-do and when abused is
considered a medical problem best handled within the doctor-
patient relationship (if considered a problem at all), while the
other abuse is associated with the underclass (or counter-culture)
and is thought by the middle and well-to-do classes as best handled by the police. Of further interest is the fact that the drug crisis has been found to be worst in the underclass. Given this, we
can appreciate the benefits of understanding abuse in the context
of a health setting rather than a law enforcement setting. In any
case, this hypocrisy is an example of social prejudice and power
and not anything else.[18]

Even as usage effects must be understood in a social context, so too must the laws and regulations that seek to contain the user's market. Pharmacological and physiological facts are mistakenly thought to be central in both cases, but such facts are trivial; the social facts are the critical facts that govern the crisis. Certainly not all the effects of usage for all the various drugs nor all the laws that govern such usage are of purely social origin. But if we were to make one clean cut through a complex and multifaceted problem, a cut intended to illuminate solutions to the problem, the cut we would make would use social and social psychological insights rather than pharmacological and physiological facts.

This then is the whole of the medicine society—pervasive general use of mood and behavioral drugs, a society that equates drug use with cure, and a society of members who routinely use drugs to maintain and enhance their lifestyle and choices. Informing the pervasive use we find a social-psychological infrastructure that is fully capable of supporting both legal and illegal use. In addition, we find active agents promoting drug use, such as Madison Avenue and professional sports programming, and government agencies actively and successfully seeking to shut down public health initiatives. We also find a certain hypocrisy covering that pervasive drug use—and laws and regulations that fully match the hypocrisy of use. Last, we find citizens, law enforcement officials, and law and policymakers in a rather profound denial of the true origin of the problem—themselves. The same people who made the crisis make the policy. Is it any wonder the policy is so flawed and ineffective?

Surely no one can capture the infinitely large and complex social fact of America. Nonetheless, it would be unnecessary mystification to claim the drug problem is beyond comprehension. If the problem of the drug crisis was made by us—and one purpose of this book is to demonstrate how—then positive action to mitigate the crisis is equally within our reach.

To make explicit the social psychology of drug use and the social-political context of the crisis does not mean that such a crisis is necessarily inevitable. To be sure, there will always be a drug problem; even if use halved, there would be a drug problem of some measure. Still, the goal remains to confine the problem as much as possible and minimize the social harm the problem can cause. Toward that end—and given that individual initiative and sensibility are the "natural healers" without which no mitigation is possible—the ultimate question is, what public action would best aid that individual initiative and sensibility?

To construct such a social policy, we must understand what drives the crisis and, equally, how it is that present policy is such a failure. What are the forces arrayed against current policy? By way of answering this, the first chapter made explicit the demand side of the drug crisis: the "medicine society."

Notes

1. Robin Room, *Alcohol and Disinhibition: Nature and Meaning of the Link*, Research Monograph No. 12. Report of a conference held 11-13 February 1981, Berkeley, CA, v.
2. Ibid.
3. Regarding marijuana and learning, an often referred to work is Howard Becker, *The Outsiders* (London: The Free Press, 1963). *See also:* Norman Zinberg, *Drug, Set and Setting: The Basis for Controlled Intoxicant Use* (New Haven: Yale University Press, 1984).
4. Barbara C. Leigh, "Beliefs About the Effects of Alcohol on Self and Others," *Journal of Studies on Alcohol* 48 (1987): 474.
5. Irene H. Frieze and Patricia C. Schafer, "Alcohol Use and Marital Violence: Female and Male Differences in Reactions to Alcohol." In *Alcohol Problems in Women: Antecedents, Consequences and Intervention*, eds. Sharon C. Wilsnack and Linda J. Beckman (New York: Guilford Press, 1984): 274.
6. By "trivial" I mean in terms of the effects discussed here. Obviously, effects such as slowed reflexes and blurred vision are critical effects if the affected person attempts to drive a car.
7. Alan R. Lang, "The Social Psychology of Drinking and Human Sexuality," *Journal of Drug Issues* 15, no. 2 (1985): 275.
8. Ibid., 284.
9. Ibid.
10. William E. Buckley, et al., "Estimated Prevalence of Anabolic Steroid Use Among Male High School Seniors," *Journal of the American Medical Association* 260 (16 December 1988): 3443.
11. Ibid.
12. Eliot Marshall, "The Drug of Champions," *Science* 242 (1988): 183-84.
13. William F. Pratt and Christine A. Bachrach, "What Do Women Use When They Stop Using the Pill?" *Family Planning Perspectives* 19 (1987): 261.
14. *American Academic Encyclopedia,* vol. 9, *Griswold v. Connecticut, 368.*
15. *ABC News Drug Abuse Poll, 1986,* ICPSR 8636. (Ann Arbor, MI: Inter-University Consortium for Political and Social Research, Spring 1988).
16. Weldon Witters and Peter Venturelli, *Drugs and Society* (Boston: Jones and Bartlett, 1988), 181.
17. David Musto, *The American Disease*, 2nd ed. (New Haven: Yale University Press, 1987), 167-75.

18. The consensual opinion I refer to can be found in David Musto, *The American Disease*, 1989; Arnold Trebach, *The Heroin Solution* (New Haven: Yale University Press, 1982); *The Great Drug War* (New York: Macmillan, 1987); Troy Duster, *The Legislation of Morality* (New York: Free Press, 1970); Alfred Lindesmith, *The Addict and the Law* (Bloomington: Indiana University Press, 1965); and in articles such as Ethan Nadelmann, "U.S. Drug Policy: A Bad Export" *Foreign Policy* 70 (1988): 83-108.

2

The Market *Internationale*

Neither individuals nor their institutions adapt easily to new conditions. Generally, it takes a crisis for individuals and institutions to appreciate the need for change. Such is the case with the drug crisis, which can be understood to be symptomatic of the more pervasive social practices and beliefs of the medicine society. In the case of the drug crisis, society is changing, but the structure of laws, attitudes, and practices has yet to adjust to the change. This factor must be given equal weight with the idea of the medicine society in order to understand how the drug crisis is being generated.

An apt comparison comes from recent American economic history, the era of "stagflation" of the 1970s. The general line of analysis, neither accepted nor argued here, is that this era of inflation and unemployment was caused by three factors: the "guns and butter" policy of the Johnson administration, the rise in oil prices created by a united oil exporters during the Nixon administration, and the declining economic competitiveness of American industry.

Regarding the latter, the general analysis runs that complacent corporate headquarters, insufficient investment in research and development, antiquated factories, and outmoded manager-employee relationships all worked together to produce goods that could no longer compete in the world marketplace (compared to earlier American successes and relative to the goods of other nations).

That international marketplace had changed with the rebirth of Europe and the rise of Asia, a change so profound that for the com-

parison we would have to go back to the nineteenth century and
the rise of American economic power. Yet American economic and
productive practices did not and would not respond to the need
for change until the pressure of the economic crisis became so
severe that, despite what we would have preferred, wrenching
change was deliberately enacted to adjust to new world conditions.

Thus, for the "stagflation" crisis of the long recession of 1971-
1982, that crisis of economic structure and practice, there is a parallel social crisis, the "drug crisis."[1] Each arose from policies that
unthinkingly executed outmoded beliefs and practices in a pro-
foundly changed world. A painful readjustment was necessary; but
in both cases, the first response, understandably, was to pursue
the familiar options that had worked well enough in the past,
options that required no deep-seated reform.

In addition, relevant to each crisis there was a particular change
that served equally to produce the crisis, in part, as well as to ren-
der the familiar remedies ineffective: the internationalization of
trade and market. This change can be labeled as the market internationale, using the very word of the prophesied, but not to be,
labor *internationale* of Marx.

Immanuel Wallerstein produced the first volume of *The Modern
World System* in 1974. Wallerstein described the beginning of this
world-system in the origins of capitalism, traditionally dated from
the sixteenth century. He argued that the outstanding feature of
capitalism is the international market; indeed, to Wallerstein, the
cross-cultural market *is* capitalism. Interpreting *World System*,
capitalism began as the market *internationale* and is continually
becoming more of what it has been from the beginning.

The expansion and intensification of international communications has been noted by any number of authors, for example,
Marshall McLuhan in *The Global Village*. Daniel Bell, in *The
Coming of the Post-Industrial Society*, points to another sort of
change, the exponential increase in contacts between peoples,
both within and across borders.[2] He cites this as the "...most striking difference...between 1798 and today."[3]

The relevant point here is this: given multiplying contacts
between peoples, the demand side of the market, or preferences,
has the means to cross borders as surely as goods. Moreover, and
directly relevant to the drug crisis, this internationalization of
preferences and markets is not limited to the legal market. The
underground market, following the wake of the legal market and

buoyed by all of the same technology, is equally an international market. Communications, transport, increased international travel, and familiarity with other lands, all the ingredients of the expansion of the international market lend themselves just as readily to an expansion of the underground market.

The expansion of international trade is a fairly routine observation, though when articles regarding it are sought in American business magazines, they are scarcely found.[4] Nonetheless, counting the trade of all nations, the value of international trade (in adjusted dollars) doubled between 1977 and 1986, a remarkable expansion for such a short time frame. A secondary feature of this internationalized market, particularly true in the capital and commodity markets, is instant internationalization, referring specifically to the immediate impact the performance of one market has upon others around the world. The instantaneousness of market communication and reaction is not itself relevant to the argument, but I forward it as a telling marker of thoroughgoing internationalization.

An example of this internationalization of markets and instant internationalization comes from the Wall Street crash of October 1987. The cause of the Wall Street crash, as to be expected, is neither universally agreed upon nor all that clear. Nonetheless, for our purposes, the point is the fact of internationalization, rather than the market event itself.[5] Whatever the reason for the crash, following the losses on the American exchange, stock prices dropped 12 percent in London, 15 percent in Tokyo and 7 percent in Toronto.[6] Likewise, in early 1990, when the Tokyo market suffered a quick and substantial decline, the Dow Jones lost 37 points on the same day. In an era of internationalization, economic events have no border.

The larger and relevant point here is that the underground market is no different from these other markets. Given an internationalized world, events in one country create effects in others. National borders, while not trivial in their consequences, nonetheless have become too small a context within which to understand national events and this includes the drug crisis.

The New York Times reported (using a State Department report as their source) an increase in underground market drug production in 1988 and reported this increase occurred "...partly because of political and economic instability in drug-producing countries...[including] civil strife in Burma, war in Afghanistan, the death of President Mohammed Zia ul-Haq in Pakistan and the declining economy in Peru."[7]

Such drug production rose despite all American attempts to thwart such an increase. Moreover, the report noted some twenty countries, all lesser-developed countries and all South American or Golden Triangle countries (the ancient poppy growing region of Afghanistan, Burma and Thailand, but also Iran, Pakistan and Laos) that were responsible for most of the world's production of illicit drugs. Such production and its rise was not due to the home market, but rather to international trade. Even as legal trade is increasing, so too is underground trade. Moreover, the American shore is a prime destination of this latter trade; 60 percent of the world's production of illegal drugs ends up in the United States.

The consequence of this internationalization is to negate, in part, the effectiveness of any law enforcement effort for such efforts must, for the most part, be confined to national borders while the active factors of the drug crisis, in this case, the internationalization of preferences and market, cross international borders.

Using cocaine as an example, the coca leaf that is destined for the U.S. market as cocaine is grown in Peru and Bolivia, refined in Colombia, and shipped to the United States, usually after a stopover in Mexico. The primary point of entry was Miami. Present evidence is that much of the action, following a federal crackdown in Miami, has shifted to Los Angeles. For Europe, Madrid, Zurich, Rome, and Copenhagen serve as the prime entry points. However, responding both to the enormous profits of the market as well as to enhanced law enforcement efforts inside Colombia, the supply routes are becoming considerably more complicated with more players seeking to share in middleman profits.[8]

Regarding the history of the supply-side, cocaine followed and utilized the paths and organization of the extensive marijuana smuggling trade that began in the 1960s. Indeed, the origins of the cocaine cartels were as marijuana smugglers. The violent cartel we now know as the Medellin cartel came about in response to pressure from M1, Colombia's left-wing guerrilla group. In 1982, responding to M1 kidnappings, various individuals involved in the cocaine trade met outside Medellin, Colombia, and formed a private army to combat M1 (eventually successfully). This was also the birth of the Medellin cartel.[9]

According to a report on one particular route, Cessna Citations and Gulfstream jets are the preferred modes of transportation to make the 3,000 mile trip from northern South America to Baja.[10] This sort of trip is made under Colombian sponsors who are bypassing the older method of selling to Mexican cartels who then turned a profit by smuggling the goods into the United States. The report estimated that some 18,000 small plane flights then ferry the cocaine into the United States. These are supplemented by any number of land-based trips across the border. Pilots are said to earn "at least" $20,000 a trip, while Mexican drivers can earn some $200 to drive a shipment across the border.[11] Peter Reuter of the RAND Corporation estimates that pilots earn not $20,000 but $250,000 for each trip. He also estimates that the average trip carries a cargo of 250 kilograms (550 lbs.) of cocaine.[12]

The jets are used to transport to the border for the obvious reason of shortening the last leg into the United States. Baja is also preferred because of its sparse population and lax or non-existent law enforcement. Regarding air transport into the United States, consider the difficulty any air patrol must have in catching such planes; even if successes were to increase, the obvious response of the smugglers would be to send empty planes as decoys across the border to harass air interdiction efforts.

There is no one route or cartel or mode of transport in this long-link production-refinement-distribution system. Various organizations at various times use whatever route is best suited for them; presumably a major factor in their choice is to find the route of least resistance. Whenever law enforcement shuts down one route, the supply organization simply shifts to another.

For example, in response to enhanced law enforcement within Colombia, there is evidence of Colombian drug marketeers switching their labs and shipment centers to Brazil. Brazil is favored for its size, including a 9,000 mile coastline, a factor that makes interdiction much more difficult. Brazil is also favored for its superior air and sea connections to the United States and Europe. Guatemala and Honduras, as well as the Caribbean, have also become significant refining and trans-shipment centers. Moreover, in these countries, unlike Colombia, government officials and the military promote the trade and make U.S. intervention much more problematic. The ironic effect of law enforcement has been to spread the profits around to new players, and hence to make the network much more diffuse and difficult to contain than before. These are examples of a new link being forged in response to law enforcement efforts. In addition, the drive to share in the profits can transform the traditional routes and connections of the trade.

For example, there is evidence that Mexico, an old link in the cocaine trade, is also becoming a refining center. Mexico has no place hospitable to the growing of cocaine, but it now refines 15 percent (Mexican government estimates) to 30 percent (U.S. estimates) of the cocaine coming into the United States. In 1985, U.S. government sources estimate that only 1 to 2 percent of cocaine was refined in Mexico. Bolivian and Peruvian sources also are making their own routes into the United States, again seeking to keep middleman and distribution profits for themselves. From a *Los Angeles Times* article: "The traffickers have an infinity of routes," according to a Costa Rican drug enforcement officer. "They are gamblers. They spread their bets all over the board. For every route we cut off, they get through on 10 others."[13]

The effect of squeezing off one pipeline is to enhance the market share of some other pipeline. The underground market by necessity and by its very nature is pluralistic, multicentered and multipronged. There just is not one center, be it a city or country or cartel or route that, if terminated, shuts down the workings of the market.

One more point: there remains the simple expediency of sending the underground market goods through legitimate sea-air cargo carriers. In fact, U.S. officials have estimated that one-half of all drug shipments enter the States through this route. There are any number of practical impediments to inspection. For example, hauling out and inspecting one closed cargo container can cost as much as $30,000. Only 3 percent of such cargo is inspected, even at this rather late date of the "war on drugs" and this represents an increase over previous inspection rates. Such shipments are further protected by port employees who work in collaboration with the drug marketeers.

Nonetheless, inspections have a short-term effect; but over the long-term, shippers skip back and forth from air to sea transport, using whatever venue is most open, or shift to another port of entry. A further factor working in the shipper's favor is the immense expansion of international trade, itself overwhelming to inspectors. At the same time, inspectors are loath to overly delay any cargo, given the outcry from the legitimate market any such delay would bring.

In part, this explains the lack of success of law enforcement in the interdiction of cocaine. Peter Reuter of RAND wrote a critical study of interdiction efforts, in which he reported that the total amount of cocaine seized by the Coast Guard and Customs Bureau has increased from 1.7 metric tons in 1981 to 27.2 metric tons in 1986 (one metric ton equalling 2,005 pounds). However, Reuter estimates that cocaine importation increased from 38-68 tons in 1981 to 111-153 tons in 1985. Hence, the growth of the trade has more than compensated for the increase in seizures. Corroborating evidence of this comes from the drop in the wholesale price of cocaine during the same time period. In fact, the price of a kilo of cocaine in 1985 was nearly half what it was in 1981 (from $60,000 in 1981 to $35,000 in 1985); hardly evidence of the effectiveness of law enforcement, even as appropriations for law enforcement were sharply increased.[14]

More current figures (for 1989) are that 160 tons of cocaine were confiscated out of a world production of 700 tons. Most (80 percent) of this production is for the U.S. market. The price is now approximately $15,000 a kilo. (As an aside here but of direct relevance later, one should understand that this is *after* $20 billion has been spent on law enforcement for the years 1986-90.) The United States has both the highest cocaine consumption in the world and the strictest laws (of comparable cultures) prohibiting its use. This adds up to a remarkable parallel to alcohol prohibition.

Reuter also examined the economics of cocaine smuggling. Perhaps the most critical (and astonishing) of his findings is that the cost of smuggling accounts for only 5 percent of the retail price of cocaine. The rest of the cost to the buyer is producer/refiner/distributor's profit. The consequence of this is that even if law enforcement agencies were able to seize, for example, one-half of all cocaine intended for the U.S. market, the effect would be to add less than 3 percent to the street price of cocaine. Moreover, given such figures, importers can afford to lose any number of shipments yet recoup all losses and produce a profit with their next successful shipment.

Reuter suspects that a prime consequence of interdiction is to drive out less-experienced smugglers and, thereby, preserve the profit of more experienced smugglers. Reuter concludes that the relative cheapness of smuggling, the adaptability of the smugglers plus the multiplicity of routes into the States make it extremely unlikely that interdiction can decrease cocaine consumption by even 5 percent. No person, either inside or outside of government, has challenged Reuter's much publicized findings.[15]

Generally, the handling of the proceeds of the underground market is marked by the same internationalization. For example, Federal agents shut down a major money laundering scheme in March 1989, an operation they called "Operation Polar Cap." Money from the sale of marijuana and cocaine were said to flow

"...from New York, Miami/Fort Lauderdale and Houston to Los Angeles, where laundered funds were sent directly to New York or through San Jose to New York and then by various routes to banks in Panama and Colombia."[16] In a separate money laundering case, a member of the Bahamas Parliament and a former cabinet officer were arrested. The Bahamas are notorious for being the home of banks that are open to the underground market as well as to the illegal or questionable banking activities of corporations in the legal market.[17]

It should not be imagined that the international aspect of the underground market in drugs is something new. Indeed, the underground market appears to have always existed in tandem with the legal market and often with the support of various governments, including the United States. Opium smuggling in the nineteenth century, for example, offers an interesting parallel to our time.

In the early nineteenth century, China was experiencing a severe drug crisis due to opium usage. The Manchu rulers made opium use illegal in 1839 and called upon those countries responsible for the trade (primarily England and the United States) to cooperate with their drug eradication program, just as we call upon and expect the cooperation of the governments of the drug-producing and distributing countries. The Chinese government wanted the right to inspect all ships coming into Chinese ports for the presence of opium cargo, hardly an extreme or unreasonable request.

Much like Colombia today, ships flying under the flag of the United States were distributors of the trade, not growers. England derived profits from both the growing of the poppy (primarily in India, under the auspices of the British East India Company) and its distribution. The U.S. government complied with the Chinese request; the English government did not. Palmerston, the British Prime Minister, gave the British response by authorizing the British Navy to seize Canton and other major Chinese ports. So began the Opium War of 1839-42. The Chinese were thoroughly defeated and signed the Treaty of Nanking, an extraordinary agreement worth examining.

The British were given (perhaps gave themselves is the better word) Hong Kong and free access to four other ports. The Chinese had to pay for all opium destroyed in the war. Furthermore, British opium traders would thereafter be subject to British laws not Chinese. In a bow to world opinion, smuggling was outlawed but opium was not specifically mentioned. World opinion was satisfied by permitting the Chinese government to keep opium illegal and British profits were protected by allowing British traders to distribute the drug in the five treaty ports. A British consul in Shanghai who affronted the delicacy of the British position by seizing three opium ships flying the British flag was removed from his post and transferred to India. In 1856, a Chinese official confiscated a cargo of opium in a British ship; the result was the second Opium War. The British prevailed again, this time successfully insisting the Chinese government make the opium trade entirely legal.

The American role in the opium trade was reduced due to the general decline of American shipping during the Civil War. After the war and throughout the latter half of the nineteenth century, a consensus emerged within the U.S. government that the opium trade ran counter to the larger interest of broadening trade with China and westernizing the Chinese people. However repugnant the latter purpose seems today, such sentiment served a good purpose by making the American government sympathetic to China's desire for international agreements that would end opium imports. Likewise, missionaries served to pressure the American government to cooperate with the Chinese and ban the trade.

The consequence of these various factors was the creation of a series of international agreements in the Hague Conferences of 1911-14. The American government was the principal orchestrator of the conferences, an example, as Arnold Taylor puts it in his classic work *American Diplomacy and Narcotics Traffic 1900-1939*, of American moralism in foreign policy producing a positive and effective end. Of course, this was also an enormous success for Chinese diplomacy, the Chinese having selected the American government as the critical Western pressure point. Following the international agreement, the United States passed the corresponding domestic legislation, the Harrison Act.[18] A tangential point here is that those who favor legalization overlook the fact that the American government has signed international treaties forbidding such legalization, even within domestic borders.

With the history of the Opium War in mind, perhaps the underground market, rather than conceived as following the development of international trade, can be understood as the spearhead of it. Moreover, we often find governments actively cooperating in aiding, rather than sealing off, such underground markets. In addition, given our own contribution to this history, perhaps we should not be surprised at this repetition in our time. The fact of the matter is that the American government both cooperates with, as well as attempts to shut down, the illegal drug trade.

For example, Manuel Noriega of Panama was known to be linked to the drug trade since 1972. However, because he was considered an important "asset" of the Central Intelligence Agency, the American government simply looked the other way until very recently.[19] Another example comes from Honduras, where Honduran military officials were reported by a DEA field agent to be involved in the drug trade. No follow-up investigation was made by the DEA. When this was brought to the attention of the chief of the DEA, John C. Lawn, he asserted that this report was no different than any number of reports received from any number of countries. Further he stated that no one had ordered him not to investigate the report, for "That would be a violation of my oath of office."[20]

However, in a reprise of the story of the British agent who turned in British opium only to be transferred for his trouble, the field office in Honduras was subsequently closed. Honduras, of course, was considered by the Reagan administration as an important anti-Sandinista ally.[21]

Likewise, Pakistan and Afghanistan officials and soldiers were known to be involved in the growing and smuggling of opium. Nonetheless, there was a deliberate decision made by the Reagan administration to ignore their participation in the drug trade, since these countries were important as anti-communist allies.[22]

Such hypocrisy may be justified in terms of overall foreign policy goals; however, it remains extraordinary given an administration that continually waves the bloody shirt of the "war on drugs." Is it any wonder that interdiction has been unsuccessful—given the government's protection of the drug pipeline? Indeed, it is incalculable just how much of the drug crisis has been produced by the government's own efforts to protect the drug trade. At other times, the Bush administration has approved or pushed for actions that were much protested by other nations. For example, in October 1989, the Bush Administration changed the laws of operation of the CIA, making it legal to approve operations that may end in the death of foreigners.[23] Likewise, the administration gave itself approval to arrest citizens or foreigners on foreign soil.[24]

One outcome of such approvals was the abduction of a Mexican national on Mexican soil in April 1990. The Mexican government has severely criticized the United States for such conduct and has threatened to withdraw law enforcement cooperation regarding the drug trade.[25] The governments we are offending are the same governments whose cooperation we are seeking in the effort to shut down non-government protected pipelines. The web of conflicting government means and priorities is becoming rather thick.

There are other sorts of straightforward examples of the limits of international action, such as the Panamanian government's resistance to U.S. pressure to tighten their banking laws and enforcement. The U.S. government claims Panama is a major center of this; the U.S.-supported government in Panama disagrees.[26]

It is not that U.S. efforts have been entirely without success (referring to efforts to crimp the pipeline and not efforts to protect it). For example, in October 1989, a major figure in the Medellin cartel was extradited from Colombia and brought to the States for trial. This was the fifth arrest of a cartel suspect and was called by federal authorities the "most important arrest and extradition from Colombia."[27] A second example of such success occurred in November 1989, when five nations froze the bank accounts (some $60 million) of a reputed drug cartel chief.[28] Most recently, the head of the Medellin cartel was arrested in 1991. Such efforts, including law enforcement efforts within the United States, will be examined in greater detail in a later chapter. The point is that the internationalization of law enforcement has little chance of succeeding, given the nature of the underground market, the backlash produced in other countries by heavy-handed law enforcement methods, and the contradictions within the policy of the U.S. government.

Nor does internationalization stop with markets. There has also been an internationalization of social problems as the social and economic problems of the underclass nations contribute to the social problem of the drug crisis here. It is the poverty of these countries that makes the drug trade attractive. This is not to say that the unemployed poor are the only ones that are involved in the underground market. The lack of opportunities in Latin America produces not only the high-living cartel chiefs and their soldiers but also the willing hands of the police officer and farmer. The farmer prefers the healthy and certain profits of the coca leaf and marijuana plant to the uncertain and meager profits from vegetables. The police officers in such countries often seek to supplement their meager income with "tips," thus making payoffs from drug marketeers part of the routine way of business.

Furthermore, the poverty of these countries combined with the impact of the profits from the drug trade can give this trade a certain legitimacy. Though the impact of the drug profits in Colombia (primarily cocaine) is not universally agreed upon, one economist estimates 20,000 to 30,000 Colombians are directly employed in the underground trade, with a total of 200,000 to 300,000 underground market-created jobs if indirect employment is counted (meaning jobs produced by the spending of underground market profits). This is in a region that suffers from a 12 percent to 16 percent official unemployment rate (the actual rate is considered higher). Indeed, until the Medellin cartel became openly violent, there was a general tolerance of the drug trade.

In Peru, the story is similar but with an added twist: drug production of the coca leaf is protected by the communist guerrillas of the "Shining Path." The coca area patrolled by the communist movement is estimated at 350,000 acres and has an annual output estimated at $1.2 billion (an estimate that appears remarkably low, given that the area is said to supply half the world's production of coca leaf). "Shining Path" does not grow the coca, rather, they protect the crops for a share of the profits. One last point—in 1988, Peru saw an inflation rate of 1,700 percent. Such a rate is only one sign of a thoroughly mismanaged economy. Such mismanagement has created tolerance and support for both the coca growers and the communist movement that protects the region's economy.

It is no accident that all of the drug-producing countries are lesser-developed; the poverty of these nations makes them especially vulnerable to profiting from the drug trade, as well as corrupting civil and police officials whose cooperation is necessary for a smooth production and distribution schedule. Moreover, the police departments of these countries should not be mistaken for the professional police departments of the United States.

The pay of a Mexican police officer, for example, is about $20 a week. In the ordinary course of business, quite apart from the underground market, police officers supplement their pay with "tips." The person stopped for a traffic violation need not go to court, the person simply pays the officer a "tip." Intersections that are particularly busy are valued, and the police supervisor is in turn "tipped" by officers for the privilege of practicing their trade at such lucrative corners. Likewise, street vendors are expected to tip the cop on the beat and failure to do so can lead to physical assault by the police.[29]

But even the use of the term "police officer" is a misnomer, for there is simply no comparison with American police. From the

Wall Street Journal, using a police source reporting on a station in Mexico City: "Officers were illiterate...and pay was so low—$60 a month—that some policemen were stealing from the factories on their beats. No one was keeping crime or payroll statistics, there wasn't even a typewriter available."[30]

Such police are police in name only. In actuality they are only another form of organized crime and this is true even without the added corrupting element of the drug trade. Further, these are the sort of police departments the U.S. government is looking to for help in stopping the drug trade. Needless to say, the government's hopes appear optimistic.

Such corruption creates the circumstances that led to the tragic death of DEA agent Enrique Carmareno Salazer in February 1985. Carmareno was successful in locating large marijuana fields in Northern Mexico and planned the raids that destroyed them. His torture and death were apparently in retaliation for the raids.[31] Nor was his the last death. In a less publicized case, DEA agent Victor Cortez was abducted and tortured in August 1986. Eleven Mexican police officers were arrested for their role in the crime. These officers were found to be an integral part of the marijuana plantation that Cortez found. For example, police officers were hired by the plantation's chief as bodyguards when he made withdrawals from banks to pay his fieldhands.[32]

It is the endemic poverty and disorganization of the lesser-developed countries, the international underclass, that creates such conditions so favorable to the drug trade. Mexico is said to be reforming its police force, but given the tremendous financial squeeze the Mexican government is under, any real solution to its combined poverty and police problem is unlikely. The United States suffers as well from the corruption of police and civil authorities. Three former DEA agents were charged with drug trafficking in November 1988.[33] A fourth was charged in August of 1989.[34] A Massachusetts prosecutor was charged with taking kickbacks from a drug marketeer in exchange for information regarding police anti-drug operations in February 1986.[35] A federal judge was convicted of taking a bribe from a drug smuggler, the first federal judge to ever be convicted of bribery.[36]

The American middle class has become corrupted as well. For example, in Los Angeles some 30 suspects, many of them jewelers, have been arrested for taking part in a money-laundering scheme. Before the arrest, police estimate that the group had "laundered" over $1 billion for drug marketeers.[37] In other words, the profit potential of the underground market in drugs tempts not only those in the underclass nations of the southern hemisphere, but is enough to tempt law enforcement agents and "upstanding citizens" in this country.

It is not as though countries such as Colombia are doing nothing. In fact, in Colombia there has been a genuine effort by the government to close down the market. Colombia has been fighting back, but with tragic results: in the last eight years 222 court workers, including 43 judges, have been assassinated by the drug marketeers. Indeed, Colombians are tiring of fighting what they call the "United States' war." Other countries are beginning to show similar resentments; Jamaica and the Bahamas are seeking United Nations troops to replace American anti-drug forces.

The international underclass has its parallel within the United States: the drug marketeers of the American underclass. The underground market in cocaine, for example, might be said to be the revenge of the American underclass. We have here the remarkable fact of the underclass of America joining forces with and creating a supply network with the underclass of South and Central America, an international (it is tempting to say "multinational") mirror image of the legal market.

How much imported cocaine can be laid at the feet of American "gangs" is controversial, as is the importance of the drug trade to the gang. The point here is that "gangs," organized crime, career criminals (by whatever name) play a certain role in the drug trade. Indeed, current policy ensures a steady and lucrative income for them. The ultimate question must be this: can law enforcement take this source of profit away from these groups?

We really should know better than to believe that the police can contain the underground market. We know that in the former USSR there exists an underground market of desired goods that are unavailable in the legal market. Consider the extensive intrusion and domination of the Soviet state over its citizens, including internal passports and no law against unreasonable search and seizures. The Soviet government (pre-*perestroika*) had the ability to monitor and regulate the everyday lives of the Soviet citizen without the consideration of the checks and balances of a decentralized Federalism, a free, even if "statehouse," press, or a Bill of Rights. Not only did they have this power, but the leaders of the Soviet Union, until Gorbachev, were fully willing to use it. Yet, the underground market survived and prospered in the Soviet Union. If social control to such a scale and degree cannot end the underground market there, how can we expect law enforcement to shut down the market here?

The Soviet Union was not able to shut down its internal market, nor was it able to shut out the rest of the world. Again, this is true despite its extraordinary power over the lives of Soviet citizens. The recent events in Central Europe can be understood as a democratic revolution and equally as a consumer revolution. The citizens of Central Europe wanted access to the same markets and goods available across the Iron Curtain. This represents an internationalization of consumer taste and preference, an internationalization that crossed the most rigid and supervised border in the world. Of course, we are no less vulnerable (indeed, far more so) and open to the same kind of internationalization, the same cross-fertilization of taste and preferences.

The problem is international, yet action across national borders is problematic. Not only is there the problem of reviving older disputes (such as between Mexico and the United States) and having such disputes interfere with the international effort, there is the problem of different cultures and different standards, for example the problem of the lack of a professional police force in many, if not all, of the countries with a hand in the cocaine trade. Then the endemic poverty of the region, combined with the poverty here, creates an army of ready recruits for the drug trade. Moreover, the profits are such that many of the middle and upper-income classes here are willing to participate in the market.

The opening paragraphs of this chapter drew a specific parallel between the drug crisis and the stagflation crisis of 1971-82. Each were said to be caused, in part, by outmoded responses to the particular crisis. In both cases, the change that rendered the responses ineffective was the same: internationalization. This internationalization helps create the market demand and the means by which this demand is supplied. Additionally, in an internationalized world, events transcend national borders; yet even when this is recognized and international action is attempted, such action is subverted by other international priorities and, quite often, the heavy-handedness of the international action.

In conclusion, the particular response to the drug crisis here has been increased police power and budgets. This has proved futile. Police action can only suppress the worst of the symptoms of social crisis, and in the case of the drug crisis, it is hard-pressed to do even that. Police action cannot touch the underlying social and economic conditions (including the internationalization of preferences and markets) nor can it produce positive change. Indeed, by ignoring such underlying conditions, the symptoms are worsened even as police action is intensified.

The advantage of the law enforcement approach is that painful and necessary readjustments can be avoided, or so it is thought, and the laws, attitudes and practices of the medicine society can go on as before, only, it is hoped, without a drug crisis. Such is the hope of those who wish to continue the status quo. Yet this response, of limited effectiveness in far more simpler times, is completely undermined by larger social changes, as well as by contradictions within itself.

Notes

1. Of course, "recession" has a technical meaning, two consecutive quarters of declining G.N.P. Here, I am using "recession" in the general sense, a protracted downturn that was something less than a "depression." "The long recession" captures, in my opinion, the long period of stagflation that began with the first oil crisis and ended in the severe downturn of 1981-82.
2. Daniel Bell, *The Coming of the Post-Industrial Society* (New York: Basic Books, 1973).
3. Ibid., 171.
4. Or such was my experience after a number of days spent in the library looking for articles in popular business magazines upon the internationalization of trade. An equally routine observation is the parochialism of American business and the lack of aggressiveness in the export market. I do not know that this is entirely true, given that American businesses continue to lead the world in exports. Nonetheless, were the Japanese or German economies the same size as ours, and their exports calculated in the same proportion, their exports would be considerably larger. In fact the Germans, with an economy approximately one-fifth the size of our own (not counting East Germany), nearly match our exports as is. The tangential point here is that the internationalization of markets is much noted elsewhere but little in American business periodicals and further, though we lead the world in exports, this is due more to the size of our economic base than the international vision of American business people.
5. "Wall Street's October Massacre," *Time*, 26 October 1987, 32-33. Yet another report blames then Treasury Secretary James Baker for making a public statement that was construed in the money market as meaning the value of the dollar was going to be deliberately driven down by Treasury. Hence any holdings in dollars would lose their value in direct proportion to the decline of the dollar, making non-dollar based investments that much more valuable. "Panic Grips the Globe," *Time,* 2 November 1987, 22-33.
6. "Wall Street's October Massacre," *Time*, 26 October 1987, 33.

7. "Drug Production Rising Worldwide, State Dept. Says," *New York Times*, 2 March 1989, I 1:3.
8. "Ingenuity of Drug Lords on the Rise," *Los Angeles Times*, 14 April 1989, I 1:1 For a more thorough account of Latin America and the drug trade see Scott B. MacDonald, *Dancing on the Volcano: The Latin-American Drug Trade* (New York: Praeger, 1988).
9. U.S. Congress, Senate Subcommittee on Narcotics, Terrorism and International Operations, *Drugs, Law Enforcement and Foreign Policy: A Report of the Subcommittee on Narcotics, Terrorism and International Operations*, 13 April 1989, 71-96. This subcommittee was headed by Senator John Kerry of Massachusetts.
10. "Southwest Connection," *Newsweek*, 23 November 1987, 29-33.
11. Ibid., 30.
12. From a prepared statement by Peter Reuter of RAND Corporation to the House of Representatives Committee on Government Operations, 17 October 1989. The statement was based upon his research performed at RAND; research requested and funded by the Federal Government. The research is Peter Reuter, Gordon Crawford and Jonathan Cave, *Sealing the Borders*, R-3594-USDP (Santa Monica: RAND Corportation, 1988).
13. "Cocaine Cuts New Routes to the North," *Los Angeles Times*, 13 April 1989, I 18.
14. From a prepared statement by Peter Reuter of RAND Corporation to the House of Representatives Committee on Government Operations, 17 October 1989.
15. Ibid.
16. "Cartel's Money Laundering Halted," Los Angeles Times, 30 March 1989. See also, "Gold, Drugs and Clean Cash," *Los Angeles Times*, 18 February 1990. This article is on the money-laundering operation centered in the jewelry district of Los Angeles. In addition, "A Torrent of Dirty Dollars," *Time*, 18 December 1989, 50-56.
17. "A Torrent of Dirty Dollars," *Time*, 18 December 1989, 52.
18. Arnold Taylor, *American Diplomacy and Narcotics Traffic 1900-1939* (Durham, NC: Duke University Press, 1969). This is considered the standard work on this topic.
19. "Fighting Narcotics: U.S. is Urged to Shift Tactics," *New York Times*, 10 April 1988, I 1:1
20. Ibid., I 10.
21. Ibid.
22. Ibid.
23. "U.S. Okays Covert Operations That May Kill Foreigners," *Los Angeles Times*, 14 October 1989, I 1:1.
24. Ibid.
25. "Mexico to Confront U.S. on Camarena Case Abduction," *Los Angeles Times*, 18 April 1990, A 1:5.
26. "Panama is Resisting U.S. Pressure to Alter Inadequate Bank Laws," *New York Times*, 6 February 1990, A 1:1.
27. "Arrest Called Key Break in Sylmar Drug Bust Inquiry," *Los Angeles Times*, 6 November 1989, A 1:1.

28. "5 Countries Freeze Drug Kingpins $60 Million," *Los Angeles Times*, 8 November 1989, A 7:1.
29. "Many Mexican Police Supplement Low Pay with Tips and Fines," *Wall Street Journal*, 25 November 1986, A 1:4.
30. Ibid., 24.
31. "Death of U.S. Agent in Mexico Drug Case Uncovers Grid of Graft," *Wall Street Journal*, 25 November 1986, A 1:1.
32. Ibid., A 1:1.
33. "3 Ex-U.S. Drug Agents Charged with I.R.S. Fraud," *Los Angeles Times*, 23 November 1988, II 1:5.
34. "A DEA Hero is Busted," *Newsweek*, 28 August 1989, 32.
35. "The Friends of David T," *Newsweek*, 10 February 1986, 68.
36. "Federal Judge Gets 6 Years in Bribe Plot," *Los Angeles Times*, 7 September 1991, A 17:1.
37. "Solid Gold Shock: Drug Money-Laundering Arrests Stun Downtown Jewelry District," *Los Angeles Times*, 24 February 1989, II 1:1.

3

The Leisure and

Personality Society

Every social fact, every sort of categorization of an era, might be proposed as being a fact rooted in the past or as something new. This is not evidence of contradiction, rather, every era can equally be conceived as the culmination of the past, a transition between that past toward some future state or as the birth of some new era. No perspective is necessarily fixed and the "right" view. What perspective is most relevant depends upon the problem at hand: in the instance of the drug crisis, all are relevant to understanding how the crisis came to be. This chapter seeks to put the drug crisis in all these lights, using writings of both the past and the present and including writings by "futurists."

American society is aptly described as a leisure and personality society as well as a medicine society. The increase in value of leisure and the importance given "personality" can be understood as something new, or as this society becoming more fully what it has long been. After all, the first description of American society as such comes from Thorsten Veblen. This chapter examines the leisure and personality society using Veblen's writings, and then examines the post-modern self and society, argued by many to be the new and distinctive social fact of our time.

The general argument regarding the impact of this social fact upon the drug crisis is the same as the arguments presented in the opening chapters. On one hand, the argument has been that the drug crisis is embedded in a larger society: the purpose of this chapter is to further define and enlarge upon those larger social factors producing and maintaining the drug crisis. This is critical to understanding why drug usage (including the problem of legal drug use) has proven to be hard to eradicate—such usage is rooted in larger social beliefs and practices.

Second, society is changing in a particular way, the infrastructure of beliefs, values, and practices is changing, yet the superstructure of law and enforcement remains unchanged. This results in the drug crisis in all of its manifestations: the primary crisis of usage as well as the secondary crisis formed by the underground market and law enforcement efforts—as present realities collide with yesterday's law.

There is another way of stating this relevant to "the leisure and personality society." The social liberalism of our time tolerates drug use; such usage is considered a matter of personal choice, even by individuals who do not themselves use alcohol/drugs. Yet the political conservatism that is equally a hallmark of our time disdains the public health approach to drug abuse and supports current laws and their enforcement. Within such contradictions, written into law and social policy, is the dynamo of the drug crisis.

Veblen, in *Theory of the Leisure Class*, perceived the beginning of new practices in American society: conspicuous leisure and conspicuous consumption.[1] Veblen placed these factors within the framework of a historical evolution of taste and power. Today, we discard Veblen's storyline: historical evolution is as out of fashion today as it was in fashion during Veblen's time. But we keep his insights as accurate predictions of what became, in time, obvious truths. Veblen wrote:

> Abstention from labor is the conventional evidence of wealth and is therefore the conventional mark of social standing; and this insistence upon the meritoriousness of wealth leads to a more strenuous insistence upon leisure...This pervading sense of the indignity of the slightest manual labor is familiar to all civilized peoples, as well as to people of a less advanced pecuniary culture...Time is consumed non-productively from a sense of the unworthiness of productive work and as an evidence of pecuniary ability to afford a life of idleness.[2]

Veblen called this "conspicuous leisure"; the twin of "conspicuous consumption." Together they defined a new era. Leisure became a status symbol (again, a phrase of Veblen's) in a land of people with no other means to differentiate their social position from others save by status symbols. Leisure, in and of itself, became prized, an emblem of wealth and success. Regarding the shunning of a productive life, Veblen was probably engaging in some hyperbolic exaggeration. Generally, Americans are supposed to be productive and will strive to give that impression, whatever the true facts of the matter.

Still, the leisure society, in which leisure is recognized as a positive value and the supply of which became a decentralized and dynamic American industry, is a fact of American society. Furthermore, this leisure activity, rather than being the domain of a particular class (such as in Veblen's time), is a movement that has filtered downward, becoming a fact of life that many (certainly not all) share.

The statistics are thus: employment in the entertainment and recreation industry has increased from 717,000 in 1970 to 1.35 million in 1987;[3] personal consumption expenditures for recreation have increased (in unadjusted dollars) from $42.7 billion in 1970 to $115 billion in 1980 to $250 billion in 1987.[4] At the same time, indicators such as attendance at sporting events, participation in sports and expenditures for sporting goods all show increases.

However, following the long recession of 1971-82, leisure time decreased and the workweek increased. In 1987, pollster Louis Harris reported that between 1973 and 1985 the number of hours spent at leisure had dropped from 26 hours to 18 hours a week.[5] As to be expected, the workweek increased by about the same amount, from 41 hours in 1973 to 49 hours in 1985. The figures for the professional class, which might be expected to be in opposition to the trend, are in fact quite identical to the overall average.[6]

Combining Harris' report of the shrinkage of leisure time and the rise in recreation, one conclusion is that Americans may have less time for leisure but have more money for it and are working in as hard and as organized a way at their leisure as they are at their work. Whatever the case, the question becomes—what is the significance of the leisure society to the drug crisis?

The point is that there has been a liberalizing trend in American society (even as there has been a trend toward political conservatism), and as this liberalizing trend includes leisure, it also accommodates alcohol/drug usage. Part of any person's leisure time is spent with friends and when friends get together for social occasions, generally a drug is produced as a token and fact of such social occasions.

Additionally, we have the element of the increase in per capita disposable income from $9,700 to $11,000 (adjusted dollars) between the years 1980 and 1987.[7] Did all Americans share in this increase? Probably not. Even as real income increased for only the upper 20 percent, so too disposable income has probably only increased for this group. Most probably, these are the true individuals fueling the drug crisis, since these are the people who have the disposable income to generate a $100 billion-a-year underground market. The underclass simply does not have the income to produce such a market. Fortunately for the upper and upper-middle income classes though, there is the underclass to take the blame and receive the brunt of police action.

Moreover, we are not only a leisure society, we are also a society of "conspicuous consumption." This is directly relevant to the drug crisis, given that cocaine consumption has always been something of a status symbol. Or, as one researcher puts it, "cocaine is the drug of the 'privileged class.'"[8] Seigel, reviewing the literature on cocaine, writes "...users seek something more than cocaine—an image of cocaine as something more than cocaine, as a privilege of the privileged. A user consumes both the drug and the image of cocaine."[9] Seigel notes that the expense of the drug itself contributes to its value as a status symbol.

In addition, we are becoming a society in which personality—the study, discussion, change, growth, fulfillment, and importance thereof—has become something of a national obsession. Though here again, this could also be understood as America becoming more of what it has always been, with the myth of the individualist and the earlier myth of America as a nation of self-fulfilled saints yielding to the twentieth century science of psychology and the internal (and external) make-over. The cult of "personality" need not necessarily mean drug usage but it could; using alcohol and/or drugs as a social lubricant, a perceived liberator and, combined with the belief in a repressed subconscious, the means by which we can experience our "true selves."

A leisure and personality society is perfectly compatible with drug usage, meaning simply that alcohol/drug usage would be tolerated in such a society, even by members who do not themselves use alcohol and/or drugs. However, this formulation is too simplistic to be left there. First of all, there is a body of writings on the "post-modern self"; a reasonable question is how this "self" might impact upon the drug crisis. Second, even as there have been increases in recreation and the use of drugs as recreation, so too there have been increases in, for example, the numbers of people attending evangelical churches. How might these social factors interact with the drug crisis? Before considering these facts, one more block of statements upon leisure follows.

Current commentators note the emergence of a new leisure class peculiar—to our time—youth. For example, consider the following quote: "The U.S. economy since the 1960's has been able for the first time to sustain a large leisure class of youngsters not in the labor force but yet consumers on a political scale or, if employed, free to spend their earnings as they please."[10] Now, a number of objections can be made to this statement (it is somewhat outdated, as it ignores those living in poverty, and most jobs available to young people are low-paying and menial), nonetheless, the fact is that many of today's youngsters are well supplied with cash and also have the opportunity to spend it on drugs.

Consider just how available illegal drugs are to youths: "86% say that marijuana is easy to get, 66% say the same for amphetamines, 55% for tranquilizers, 51% for barbiturates, 49% for cocaine, 31% for LSD, 26% other psychedelics, 21% for heroin, and 33% for other narcotics, including methadone."[11] These statistics concern high school seniors. The locales from which Harris is drawing his data are somewhat unclear.

Nonetheless, other research on even younger people and from locales that are decidedly middle-class, report equally alarming facts. For example, one survey of sixth to eighth graders conducted in 1986 reported that 1 percent of sixth graders reported trying heroin, 2 percent LSD, 3 percent cocaine, 3 percent amphetamines, 6 percent inhalants, 11 percent marijuana and 65 percent alcohol. The data was drawn from two middle-class, middle American small towns.[12] What does this mean?

The point is not that youth, of whatever age, are responsible for the drug crisis. Drug usage peaks, population-wise, in the late twenties (with all sorts of variation, given ethnicity and gender).[13] Nonetheless, the existence of the youth market creates another dimension to the drug crisis, a dimension that did not exist during the alcohol prohibition of 1920-1933. Particularly problematic regarding efforts at mitigation is the economic power of this new culture; it has both the means and the ability to mimic adult culture, including indulging in drug usage.

"New youth culture" here does not mean youth culture in general. There has been such a thing probably since the 1920s and possibly since the founding of the modern university system in the

1890s. What is continually "new" is the diffusion of this youth culture down to increasingly younger age groups. For evidence of this, consider that fashion designers and clothes outlets now gear up for a 10- to 12-year-old market, a market that did not exist in previous eras. This age group has disposable income, is actively appealed to by the legitimate market and, as to be expected, has access to and uses illegal drugs. The creation of such a market is a new social fact, and 10- to 12-year-olds participating in the underground market is a new factor in our "drug crisis."

To make the point about the drug crisis and current policy—even as the narrow-minded perspective of the law enforcement option must be rejected as self-defeating (and not a little hypocritical), still the concerns of those who sincerely put forward that option must be understood in the context of concern over young people's use of drugs. However mistaken their support for current policy, their concerns are genuine and easily understood. Secondly, regarding the present focus upon cocaine as the demonized drug of evil, even if cocaine usage were entirely eliminated, there are plenty of other drugs available to young people. The elimination of one drug would only lead to the increased use of some other equally available drug. We must go deeper into the social fabric if we are sincere in our concern for the health of our young people.

The Post-Modern Self and Society

There has been a voluminous amount of writing about the profound difference between our age and previous eras, writings that stress a profound break between them. Exactly what has changed is subject to any number of formulations: the "computer age" (Berkeley 1962), the "post-modern society" (Etizoni 1968), the "information age" (Helvey 1971), the "post-industrial society" (Bell 1973), the "communications age" (Phillips 1975), and the "third wave" (Toffler 1980) are a handful of examples. Whatever the specifications of the change, all authors tend to note the same kinds of things, so a certain broad outline of change can be distilled from these diverse sources.

Daniel Bell perceived a "post-industrial society" in which he noted what has become a cliche: the transformation of the economy into a service-orientated economy, the rise of the suburbs and the emergence of a youth culture. The latter two features are possibly outdated hallmarks of the past, though it seems that the importance of cities is not as diminished as we might think and that the

importance of the youth culture of the sixties proved transitory—
at least as a political force.

Nonetheless, Bell fit into the general sort of argument usually
made regarding our time when he noted the machine and the factory were receding in central importance and being replaced by
information and knowledge. These were the new fulcrums of the
age, the new agents of change and the heart of the new order. This
latter idea is first found in Amitai Etizoni's work, *The Active
Society* (1968). Etizoni, writing before Bell, introduced the notion
of "post-modernity." Etizoni's vision, even as it predated Bell,
went somewhat beyond Bell's perspective. The new world was not
an extension of the old in any significant way but a new era in and
of itself. Etizoni's key word, to remarkably and perhaps even
unfairly simplify his work, was "knowledge."

Knowledge equalled power in Etizoni's argument. He did not
mean coercive power but rather a genuine empowerment of individuals and their society to deliberately effect change. There was no
dynamic that would inevitably produce positive change but the fact,
according to Etizoni, that distinguished this new society was the
dynamic of change itself—the power of individuals and their society to produce change—in whatever direction. Communications and
technology were subsumed under knowledge. To Etizoni, they were
a form of knowledge themselves and a transmitter of other forms of
knowledge.

This is quite relevant to the present crisis. Applying Etizoni to
the "drug crisis," we can understand that contradictions between
practice and law are possibly going to have a greater impact than
in previous ages and that there may be a greater price to pay for
such contradictions as communications (simply "knowledge" to
Etizoni) that reverberate within and across borders and between
countries as quickly as between friends in the coffeehouse. Events
can spin out of control that much easier and quicker. There also
appears a greater potential for deliberate social change. The same
technology that makes possible "crisis" is the same technology
that makes possible deliberate change—that is, were policy
enacted on the basis of dispassionate analysis and not prejudice
and the need for re-election.

Alvin Toffler, in *The Third Wave* (1980), following the general
wisdom, wrote of the computer/communications/technology age
in terms of an evolution from the agricultural revolution to the
industrial revolution to the third revolution of the computer.
Historical scenarios of social evolution are reassuring in that they

console us that progress is being made, but current thinking considers "progress" and "evolution" the key words of the Victorian era and, however commonsensical, difficult to specify when all the facts are considered. Nonetheless, within Toffler's argument there are telling points relevant here.

Toffler argued that "mainstream culture" is a myth. He argued that the "mainstream" has disintegrated, fractured into numberless subcultures. The least of these subcultures is based upon ethnicity, the conventional understanding of subcultures. Rather, subcultures include, for example, the youth culture, new movements such as feminism, gay and lesbian liberation, the "moral majority," new wave, environmentalism and so on. Rather than being born into a subculture such as ethnicity, the distinctive fact of our time is that as individuals we are free to choose the subculture of our choice. Alongside the market of economy, there is the market of culture, with individuals able to pick the culture that best suits them.

One must understand, were this true (and it certainly appears so), the difficulty any law would have in governing such a culture. There are many cultures of varying values and norms but there can be only one law. This suggests that rather than taking a hard-nosed approach to the law, we would further social peace by appreciating the cultural pluralism of our time and write law that accommodates, rather than suffocates, pluralism.

Furthermore, Toffler appears to argue that integration is occurring, but at the level of the individual (another facet to the cult of personality) and their small social groups rather than at the "mainstream." The individual, to Toffler (and this is my interpretation of Toffler; he did not write this directly), is re-emerging from the "lonely crowd" of Riesman (1961), and they are doing so by both "finding themselves" and by finding the social group, the subculture, with which they can identify. These subcultures too can be understood as "new cultures," though what may be genuinely "new" is the recognition of such.

Relevant to the purpose of this work, drug usage and the underground market is as much a manifestation of these larger changes as is the computer. An old consensus on the preference of alcohol and tobacco over all other drugs is breaking down as surely as are other sorts of conventions. The "post-modern self" is likely to look to itself and to small social groups for cues as to what is acceptable or unacceptable behaviors. As such, purely legal strictures are likely to be ignored, as is the case today.

The Neo-Victorians

In regard to the term post-modern self, it is not to be imagined that this describes everyone or even nearly so, but it does not have to. Whatever the number of persons it describes, the more critical factor is that such people support a $100-billion-a-year industry. And when the drug preferences of the rest of the population is included—another $100-billion-dollar-a-year industry—the outcome is a market greater than all, save housing, medical care, the oil industry and the auto industry.

How might the rest of the population be described? An apt word might be *neo-Victorian*. As noted, a society in any given time can be understood as something being born, in terms of the future, but a society can also be understood in terms of becoming what it has long been. Given that the subject is American society, this means a Victorian society. We generally use the word "Puritanism," but history is often more recent than we think and, in my opinion, Victorianism is the more accurate term.

Now as then, there is the same anxiety over what appears (and is) accelerating turbulence combined with the same rigid public front that nothing really has changed. In other words, the attitude is that there is no need for fundamental reform, or that the world may have changed but there is no need for the law to, nor any need to change our understanding of government and what "governing" means. To the Victorians, government was sensibly restricted to the police and the various municipal services. Social tensions and ills such as poverty were best met with the tools at hand—the police.

This is the case today as well. And the picture is complete with Victorian admonitions of the need for family values in response, for example, to the problem of children's malnutrition and lack of health care. The problem resides within families, the Victorians maintained, and like today, they were generally referring to families of a particular sort, the minorities of their era: the Irish, Italians and Jews. Of course, the Jewish-Americans escaped the blame for crime and poverty. Instead they were given a more ominous burden—responsibility for an international communist conspiracy. As in the earlier heyday of Victorianism, even anti-Semitism is reviving in our time. One more parallel is that the first cocaine crisis occurred in the Victorian era at the turn of the century.

Generally, we have forgotten just how anxious these people were. Religion was under attack, faith purported to be a matter of

delusion, evidence of a psychological need for security and sub-
mission to a father figure. Similarly, there was a great fear of com-
munism (the first Communards came into existence in 1830 and
1848). We have been fearful of the "red menace" for a long time.
The machine and factory were king, but the unparalleled production of goods was just as equally matched by the extraordinary
numbers of the poor and the depth of their poverty. The values
and world view of the Victorians were under attack on all fronts.
Indeed, the undermining of those values by new conditions combined with the rigidity of the response is Victorianism.

Nonetheless, the original Victorians had another side as well.
Public education was valued; the modern university system was
born; the world's first public health system and public transportation system were built. All these were created by these Victorians.
Moreover, even as their homes were built to last, their public systems, their schools and their transportations systems were the
finest of the age. In addition, they designed their small towns as
villes; they never forgot that they lived in a community. Today's
neo-Victorians should blush.

Regarding how many people might be so described, the more
critical point is that they have carried the day—their opinion is
law. The law labels all non-mainstream drugs as "narcotics" and
threatens to place 20 percent of the population—as a beginning—
behind bars, even if it means every violent repeat offender
presently in jail has to be released back to the street. Not surprisingly, given the enormity of the task of imprisoning the 20 percent
of the population that rejects mainstream drugs of choice, the law
enforcement option has run into some difficulty achieving its task
and the drug crisis continues.

The question becomes: who are the neo-Victorians and who are
the post-moderns? Are they like two armies locked in some sort of
mortal combat? Newspaper headlines, given the journalistic preference for he/she versus him/her type storylines, might lead one to
think of the world in such a way. But in fact the groups that have
the attention of the press represent relatively small, though influential, numbers.

It could well be that there are particular individuals aptly
described by such labels. But it is also likely that such categoriza-
tions exist within individuals, contradictions and all. This would
make sense, in my opinion, given that we experience and are
socialized into the world as it is, with all its contradictions.
Moreover, consistency is a virtue of the inventions of philosophy

and mathematics; in the natural human universe, inconsistency and paradox are the general rules. For most if not all of us, when our opinions are examined in their entirety, we find elements of the new, the post-modern, as well as the old, the Victorian.

The conflict is more usefully understood—not as between groups of people so much as between action and word. From the same population that consumes 60 percent of the world's production of illicit drugs[14] and spends some $170 billion on licit and illicit behavioral drugs also comes the world's most rigid drug laws (of comparable cultures). Such a fact describes a population in collective denial.

Conservative laws are doomed to fail when accepted social practice is so liberal. Nonetheless, it should not be thought that the problem is only about law (though ultimately, the law is critical). There have been previous periods of conservative reaction, but also previous eras of overall liberal attitudes (most recently, the 1970s). What kept liberal attitudes from being translated into law was the fear of addiction, or more accurately, the inability of therapists to "cure" it. The concerns of those who favor rigid laws are genuine and must be given their due, both in the matter of addiction and the concern over young people's use of drugs.

However, if we want to effectively attack the problems of addiction and young people's drug use, the most appropriate way is through reform, both of the law and of social policy. Exhortations of values will not work in either the medicine society or the leisure and personality society—for drug usage is completely consistent with the values of this society. Nor will the recourse to police work when exhortations fail. As an example we have the 1920s, another era in which rigid law was matched to liberal practice, and our own era is rapidly becoming another example of failure. Nor can we point to some era when drug laws worked—the fact is Americans have always had liberal alcohol/drug practices. If we are sincere in our concerns over the problem of drug usage and the harm irresponsible individuals (whether addicted/alcoholic or not) cause others, we are going to have to reach for genuine reform. Present action is simply taking the easy way out.

A considerable amount of time has been spent presenting the subtleties of the current writing about our era and applying that writing to the drug crisis. However, for the sake of presenting all the facts, there is a simpler explanation that could substitute for all these words and that explanation is this: Americans are simply not a particularly law-abiding people.

When Lyn Nofziger, a special assistant to Ronald Reagan, was indicted for influence peddling his reply was twofold. First of all, he complained, the law was bad and what he did should not be considered against the law. Secondly, he did not do anything different than anyone else—everyone was doing it.[15] Eventually, an appeals court agreed and threw out a jury verdict.

Mr. Nofziger's reply was typically American, an opinion any number of us have shared at one time or another. Moreover, over 100 officials of the Reagan administration were indicted on some charge or another. One official, Oliver North, convicted of lying to Congress, became a hero. In other words, consistent with our frontier disdain for the law, we, as a people, see no great evil in breaking the law. The one condition is that no one is directly and physically harmed by another. Otherwise, law-breaking is not considered such a terrible thing—though we could never say so publicly. This Americanism must be set alongside the more elaborate arguments previously presented.

To summarize the main points; the conspicuous leisure and consumption that Thorsten Veblen defined is just as much a fact of America as ever, with the sole exception being that such values have extended to include more sorts of people than the descendants of American patricians. Alcohol and drug use is perfectly compatible with this American mindset. Americans are at the same time neo-Victorians, happy with their moralistic frame and determined to use the police as an adjunct clergy responsible for putting people on the right path or, that failing, functioning as the arm of punishment when the people stray. In this way, a useful example is made for the rest of the population regarding the consequences of deviance. This is the thinking that constructs American drug laws and policies. Liberal practice is joined with conservative law and the outcome is the "drug crisis" in all its forms.

Liberal practice is further extended in the "post-modern" society. This is a description of a society in which the mainstream is fractured, more myth than real, with members more truly described as living within their small, self-selected subcultures. Such members look to their subcultures rather than law or custom for guidance in values and practice. American society is thus multicultural and has a number of dimensions. Flexible law is called for but the traditional response of more law and greater penalties is being exercised. In this way, we can understand the drug crisis has deeper and broader roots than drug practices and policies per se.

In the next chapters, two sorts of institutionalized agents of social control will be examined: the public health system and law enforcement. How are these agencies doing in the "war against drugs"? Each, rather than contributing to the containment of the problem, have instead aggravated the problem. Public health is crippled by declining funding and previous funding was not generous or extensive in scope. The law-enforcement effort is caught in a great paradox and plagued by its own inconsistencies. The next section seeks to make the case for this argument. In addition, the research upon drug usage, treatment and education will be covered.

Given the argument of the failure of the public health and law enforcement systems to control the crisis, the question becomes: what is containing the problem?

Notes

1. Thorstein Veblen, *The Theory of the Leisure Class* (New York: Mentor, 1953 [1899]).
2. Ibid., 44-46.
3. Bureau of the Census, *Statistical Abstract of the U.S.: 1989,* No. 645 (Washington, DC: U.S. Government Printing Office, 1989), 391.
4. Bureau of the Census, *Statistical Abstract of the U.S.: 1989,* No. 377 (Washington, DC: U.S. Government Printing Office, 1989), 221.
5. Louis Harris, *Inside America* (New York: Vintage, 1987).
6. Harris notes that there might be a confounding variable here, the increase in number of women in the workforce. From the data given, it is unknown how much the effects of this factor produces the raw data quoted in the text.
7. U.S. Bureau of the Census, *Statistical Abstract of the U.S. 1989,* No. 693 (Washington, DC: U.S. Government Printing Office, 1989), 426.
8. Ronald K. Seigel, "Cocaine and the Priviledged Class," *Advances in Alcohol and Substance Abuse* 4 (Winter 1984): 37-50.
9. Ibid., 38.
10. *The New Encyclopedia Britannica, 15th ed.,* s.v. "Social Differentiation."
11. Harris, *Inside America,* 78.
12. Katherine Grady, et al., "The Emergence of Adolescent Substance Abuse," *Journal of Drug Education* 16 (1986): 203-19.
13. National Institute of Drug Abuse (NIDA), *Drug Use Among American High School Students, College Students and Other Young Adults— National Trends Through 1989* (Washington, DC: U.S. Government Printing Office, 1989).
14. U.S. Congress, Senate Subcommittee on Narcotics, Terrorism and International Operations, *Drugs, Law Enforcement and Foreign Policy* (Washington, DC: U.S. Government Printing Office).
15. "Nofziger Resentful on Eve of Ethics Violation Trial," *Los Angeles Times,* 11 January 1988, I 1:1.

Part Two
The Failure of Mitigation

4

The Crisis in Public Health

The drug crisis is embedded in the medicine society, the leisure and personality society, and the fact of market internationalization, but that is only half the story. The drug crisis is also an outcome of the failure to make a commitment to public health and the decision to focus resources on the law enforcement. This is the essence of the argument presented here.

It is the combination of these two sets of social facts that has produced the drug crisis. They are also combined in a particular way: the medicine society, the market *internationale* and the postmodern society are the factors generating the drug crisis, while the public health system, the institution that should be providing prevention and treatment care to alleviate the crisis, is itself in crisis. American society suffers from a poverty of public health and one way it suffers is the presence of a drug crisis.

Moreover, law enforcement, the other would-be mitigator, is saddled with conflicting policy demands, turf competition, and the failure of leadership to establish priorities. Hence, the worst of both worlds is produced. Law enforcement has proved unable to effectively cut down the supply side, while the creation of an underground market has brought with it all the usual effects: official and honest-citizen corruption and collusion with the market. This will be made explicit in the following chapter.

The reason the public health system is in crisis is no mystery. The first cause is the meager funding that represents an utter lack of commitment to create a first-rate health system. The second is the lack of a true national system: instead the American people are ill-served with layers of uncoordinated and disparate bureaucracies, each competing against all for their share of what funding exists.

All agencies of public health are plagued by funding shortages. Many agencies are equally plagued by uncertain funding, not knowing from year to year (or month to month) if their funding will be continued. The entire system (though, of course, there is no real system as such, more an uncoordinated and in-debt conglomerate) suffers from crisis management. Americans invented modern business economics for the rest of the world but no such rational principles (such as planning, organization and the consideration of the opportunity costs of not having a public health system) ever seem to get applied to public health.

According to an editorial in the *New England Journal of Medicine* some 40 million Americans have no health insurance at all.[1] This is true despite the fact that approximately 11.5 percent of the gross national product is spent on health care.[2] In an article by Arthur J. Barsky, the situation was described as "...a paradox of excess and deprivation;" $465 billion was spent on health care in 1986, yet for so many there is no health care at all.[3] These are the people who do not receive medical benefits at work, cannot afford to buy their own, and are not covered by Medicare or Medicaid. They are the people who fall through the cracks between public aid and private health plans and they comprise 16 percent of the American population.[4]

Moreover, there are particular segments of the population that disproportionately comprise that 17 percent of the population: mothers and children. Some 26 percent of women of child-bearing age do not have health insurance, meaning there will be no prenatal care for their infants. Such statistics contribute to the grim infant mortality rate of the United States. One in ten American babies dies before his or her first birthday. The United States ranks nineteenth among industrialized countries in infant mortality. "The safety net just isn't there for children," Rae Grad, director of Congress' National Commission to Prevent Infant Mortality, is quoted as saying.[5]

These figures represent averages. In poorer neighborhoods, infant mortality is much worse. The Children's Defense Fund reported in 1984: "The nonwhite infant mortality in our nation's capital exceeds that in Cuba and Jamaica, both significantly poorer countries. Statewide data mask more severe infant death problems in some city neighborhoods. For example, two Baltimore census tracts show infant death rates as high as 59.5 per 1,000 live births.

This exceeds the 1981 infant death rates in Costa Rica, Panama, Guyana, and Trinidad and Tobago and is more than double the rates in the Soviet Union."[6] The non-white infant mortality rate is about twice as high as the white infant mortality rate. However, the white infant mortality rate would still only rank ninth worldwide.[7]

The lack of pre-natal care contributes to such ignominious statistics. The Reagan administration, defending its cutback in funding for pre-natal programs, claimed that smoking, drinking, and drugtaking by pregnant women cause infant mortality.[8] But health experts maintain that it is a lack of pre-natal care and the malnutrition of many mothers that are the critical factors generating such shameful mortality statistics. The one segment of the population we should not want to sacrifice to budget cuts and/or military expenditures are mothers and children. Yet the programs many depend on are often the first cut.

The problem is larger than the lack of health care per se. According to an article appearing in *Scientific American* on the problem of infant mortality: "Frequently the babies weigh less than 2,500 grams (5.5 pounds) at birth because of the mother's poor nutrition."[9] There is a direct correlation between the size of babies and their chances of survival in the first year.[10] Further, there is a direct correlation between infant death mortality and the poverty of the mother or parents. Unfortunately, Federal food-assistance has not been increased. Rather, food programs have been cut back by $12 billion (unadjusted for inflation) during the 1980s.

Such cutbacks have also affected school-age children. The school lunch program, for example, was cut by $5 billion between 1982 and 1985. The effect of such cutbacks has been the reappearance of hunger, a word incapable of being precisely defined but pragmatically defined as "chronically short of the nutrients necessary for growth and good health."[11] Hunger had been virtually eliminated in the 1970s, but with the budget cutbacks it is now estimated that some 12 million children and 8 million adults, about 9 percent of the population, suffer from hunger.

Returning to health care, the National Association of Children's Hospitals and Related Institutions issued a report in 1989 calling attention to the routine lack of health care for many children.[12] They estimate that 7 million children receive no health care at all, that 60 percent of children under the age of four have not received basic immunization, as well as noting that the incidence of children with AIDS has doubled (from 10,000 to 20,000 reported cases) and that reported deaths from child abuse has increased 23 percent from 1985 to 1986. The article was based upon a report from the National Association of Children's Hospitals and Related Institutions released March 1, 1989.[13]

Estimates vary, but using data from a congressional commission on infant mortality, some 18 million children under the age of 13 are not covered by public aid or a private health plan. Yet no money has been allocated by the Federal government to deal with these new problems. The experts warn: "Quite simply, our social and political negligence is creating generations of medically home-less children, for whom we will all pay a very high price in the years to come."[14]

But this is not a matter for the future: the consequences (such as violent "gangs") are obvious now. No doubt as these problems con-tinue to hit home, the claim will be made that we remain in the throes of a "drug crisis" or a "crime wave." Such a diagnosis may be a comfort to the public and their politicians but such claims become self-fulfilling prophesies as fundamental reform is put off in favor of more law enforcement.

Criminologists tell us the incidence of crime peaks at age 15, and this is a statistic generally true across cultures and across time. When many American adolescents become 15, they do so after an upbringing without health care and, for many, without even ade-quate nutrition. Certainly there should be parents looking after such adolescents and certainly there is a failure of family respon-sibility when young people go without health care and food. But there is equally a failure in the society, in social responsibility as well as parental responsibility, when so many young people go without such essential needs. Such conditions are cultures for criminal behavior, with or without drugs.

This is not to excuse the behavior of any individual. A "society" fails to make sense when individuals are no longer held responsi-ble for their conduct. This is true whether the individuals are priv-ileged individuals who control the actions of financial institutions, government officials in positions of high trust, or minority teenagers.

There are still other consequences. The squeeze of declining reimbursements from federal programs and growing numbers of individuals without health insurance has put many hospitals on the financial ropes, particularly those that serve the poor. In 1986, hospitals nationwide lost $7 billion caring for those without health insurance. This can be compared to the $2.8 billion lost in 1980 (inflation adjusted dollars).

Responding to the crisis, the Reagan administration proposed a $7 billion cut in Medicare and Medicaid expenditures. Similarly, for 1990, the Bush administration recommended a cutback of $8 billion. But hospitals and doctors, before the cut was proposed, have complained that they are not adequately reimbursed for expenses, that payments are routinely late by months and, at times, not forthcoming at all. Hospitals in particular blame the deficit in reimbursement as a leading cause of their current fiscal crisis.

For example, the day after the state of Illinois ran out of Medicaid money (in 1987), Mary Thompson Hospital of Chicago, a hospital with 80 percent of its patients on public aid, was forced to close its doors.[15] The next year, a second Chicago hospital, with a similar caseload of indigent patients, followed suit. Overall, some 79 hospitals closed their doors across the country in 1987.[16]

Some of those that stay open do so by cutting back on staff and equipment; in other words, by cutting back on the quality of patient care. They have little choice. One expert, speaking of Roseland Hospital in Chicago, a hospital forced to cut back on care to stay open, described Roseland in a way that could fit all such hospitals: "The hospital is suffocating. These hospitals need nurture. As long as you look to marketplace solutions, you will have Roselands closing down."[17] This statement is from Dr. Quentin Young, president of the Health and Medicine Policy Research Group.

Though inner-city hospitals with high numbers of patients without insurance plus high numbers of patients with only Medicaid or Medicare are hardest hit, still: "All hospitals are dramatically feeling the Medicare squeeze," according to Linda Miller, president of the Volunteer Trustees of Not-For-Profit Hospitals and chief lobbyist for more than 3000 voluntary, non-profit hospitals. "It's universal."[18] This opinion is seconded by Dr. Thomas Frist, chairman of the Hospital Corporation of America. He has stated: "It is estimated that more than 50 percent of all U.S. hospitals will lose money on their Medicare business in 1989."[19]

Government officials dispute this. Glenn M. Hackbarth, deputy administrator of the Health Care Financing Administration, replies in regards to hospital closings: "In the next 5 to 10 years, we can do with fewer hospital beds than we have today. The hospital industry operates at an average occupancy rate in the low 60's. We don't need as many hospitals as we have right now."[20]

What this analysis overlooks is that inner-city hospitals are desperately needed, yet they are the first to close their doors. Not only that, if nothing is done about the underlying cause of hospitals closing their doors, when will the closings stop? Hospital closings are presented by such administrators as a solution to the fiscal crisis of hospitals, but if hospitals lose money on each Medicare/Medicaid patient, simply increasing the percentages of beds occupied will not solve their fiscal crisis, but will worsen it.

The hospital crisis is general, in the sense that many hospitals have become underfunded, but it is also specific. For example, care units such as obstetrics and the emergency room appear to have been particularly hard hit by the problems reported above. In a Los Angeles area county hospital, one group of doctors in the obstetrics unit decided to tape their typical night so that county supervisors would have a first-hand look at the consequences of underfunding. The resulting film had the desired effect: funding was increased to handle the 25 percent patient overload.[21]

A local solution was found there but the problem is national. Private hospitals are willing to take on public patients, but many are willing to take only obstetric patients and not others. This is contrary to federal regulation, whereby a hospital cannot pick and choose what sort of care it will provide at Medicare rates. However laudable federal policy may be here, perhaps an exception is called for, given the general demand and drain upon public hospitals.

Within the hospital crisis, there is yet another aspect to the crisis in public health, a funding crunch in the emergency room. In Los Angeles, a number of hospitals have closed their emergency rooms due to escalating costs and declining payments. California Medical Center threatened in May 1988 to close their emergency room because of continuing financial losses, primarily from the emergency care of those without health insurance. Many experts feared this would mean the collapse of the remaining emergency care system in Los Angeles. However, a last minute agreement by county and state health officials to pump more money into the system convinced the Medical Center to reverse their decision.[22]

Nonetheless, the Center's president declared: "Shoring up a crumbling health care financing system with piecemeal solutions, or propping up one strategically located institution is like putting a Band-Aid on a major hemorrhage."[23] California is not the only place where this is a problem. In Dade County, Florida, only 10 out of 30 hospitals are admitting emergency patients because of soaring expenses (including malpractice insurance expenses) and meager reimbursements.[24]

Such circumstances are part of the larger problem of emergency care. According to one estimate, out of some 142,000 deaths each year due to trauma (trauma is the leading cause of death for the population under age 34), some 25,000 deaths are preventable.[25] The problem is inadequately funded and under-staffed emergency rooms. In addition, there is the problem of the location of emergency rooms.

According to recommendations by the American College of Surgeons, a national network of 350 trauma centers could be established that would put every American within 20 minutes of help.[26] Timing is critical, as the first hour after injury is pivotal to providing restorative care. Yet only 50 such centers exist and much emergency care is administered by non-experts in facilities that are trauma centers in name only. The result, according to Dr. Kenneth L. Mattox of Houston's Ben Taub General Hospital: "Millions of injured are made worse by improper care."[27]

In another area of health care, mental health care, the story is the same: a crisis in public health. A group of California psychiatrists issued a statement they called "a declaration of conscience."[28] Condemning the latest round of cuts in mental health expenditures they stated: "Very few people who need treatment get it, and for many the treatment they receive is questionable at best."[29] This statement refers to the situation existing prior to the budget cuts of 1989 and 1990.

Regarding the state of affairs prior to the cuts, the experts noted that San Diego County refuses to admit nine out of ten people seeking voluntary hospitalization and in Los Angeles County a proposed cut will close eight outpatient clinics. The psychiatrists described a statewide condition in which "...the gravely disabled are most often treated in the emergency room and sent away on the same day."[30] The funding of the Los Angeles clinics remained a political football, with stories of funding found and funding lost alternating throughout the year and continuing so up to the time this manuscript went to press. Such uncertain funding is a typical story and is another aspect of the public health crisis.

AIDS has received considerable attention in the media. It should come as a surprise to no one that the number of individuals suffering from AIDS is increasing. Yet programs designed to help such sufferers are reducing their efforts because of the lack of funding. In Los Angeles, a program called AIDS Project Los Angeles has cut five staff positions and reduced all staff salaries by 5 percent to deal with cutbacks in both private contributions and governmental grants. This cutback is occurring despite the increase in clients from 740 in 1986 to 1,800 in 1988 and an expected doubling in 1989.

Similarly, there has been considerable media attention on the problem of rape. What has gotten less attention is the fact that funding for programs designed to aid rape victims are, once again, being cut. A good example of this is the history of the Rape Crisis Center of Santa Barbara, California. The center lost much of its funding in 1981 when many social programs were cut at the Federal level to pay for the defense buildup. The center lost 75 percent of its funding that year. The center mans a 24-hour hotline and offers a variety of services (in addition to counseling) such as self-defense classes and even accompanying victims to the hospital and/or police station. The center even trains professionals such as police officers, social workers, teachers, and others in how to help the victim of rape. This is the only program in this town (population 80,000) that offers such services. Yet workers there often do not know from month to month whether they will be paid and the center is constantly on the verge of having to close its doors. According to the director of the program: "We have been operating on basically the same budget for the past five years." This is true despite a doubling of the work load.

Directly relevant to the drug crisis is the lack of adequate funding for drug treatment centers. In New York, state officials estimate that there are some 250,000 heroin addicts in the state and some 270,000 heavy cocaine and "crack" users. Officials in New York City, however, estimate that there are some 600,000 cocaine and crack abusers in the city alone. However, in the entire state, there are only 47,000 treatment slots. Who is to pay for adding more slots? City and state officials point to each other. One state official remarked: "Municipalities have a responsibility to try to match us dollar for dollar. It's easy for somebody to point the finger and say the state isn't doing enough. But the truth of the matter is that nobody's doing enough."[31]

Curious "catch-22" situations can arise from the lack of drug treatment programs. A story from Santa Barbara County in California illustrates the problem. Offenders convicted of crimes related to their drug abuse are required to be enrolled in a treatment program in order to be released from jail. However, there are hardly any such programs to be found in the county or in neighboring counties. Therefore, the offenders stay in jail. It is like telling them to "...take a train to Hawaii," a member of the county parole board put it. "They can't fulfill that obligation because there are...no facilities available."[32]

The story is the same across the country. In a study reported on in the *Los Angeles Times*, researchers posing as addicts seeking help from treatment programs or hotlines failed 40 percent of the time to get on the programs' waiting lists or to even get an appointment. Quite often the information they were given was erroneous. Even if successful in getting on a waiting list, clients generally wait three months before receiving treatment. Moreover, a frequent condition is that they are actively addicted, if an addict stops using drugs, he or she is ineligible for help. Overall, treatment slots in Los Angeles County have declined, from 5200 publicly funded slots in 1982 to 5,170 this year. Moreover, the combination of rising costs and static funding has resulted in a decline in the numbers of people receiving help via those slots, from 23,000 in 1982 to 15,000 this year.[33]

In Boston, there is a school called the Maurice J. Tobin school and it is typical of the inner-city school.[34] When asked, a third of the children will respond that they have not had breakfast. A teacher can tell a story of a youngster who saw her mother stabbed 18 times. Another, a five year old, is kept home by a drug-addicted mother to help care for children who are even younger. Another child was dropped off at school even though suffering from an asthma attack. Yet another child attempts to hide a knife wound. In the playground, the children at one time had to be warned not to pick up the needles discarded by addicts and dealers.[35]

"What we find is people emphasizing how distressing things were at home and how unsupportive the home environment was, using this to rationalize how destructive the school environment can be," states Joseph Grannis, professor of education at Columbia University's Teachers College and a person with hands-on experience at schools like Tobin. He then adds: "While I can agree about how distressing these situations are for kids, for many of them school still is a place of hope."[36]

Indeed, the teachers at the Boston school know of students who dread summer, for it robs them of the one security in their life, school. The principal at Tobin persevered and, by allowing police to use the classroom as a lookout, was able to get the dealers out of the playground. Over the summer, the classroom was firebombed in retaliation. Nonetheless, the school hung tough and the dealers had to move. For such determination, there is precious little help or encouragement coming from the city, state, or Federal government. At one time, there was a full-time student support worker to help coordinate with social workers. Now, due to budget cutbacks, there is no aide. Further, the principal of this school had her salary cut this year.[37]

Even as the public health crisis becomes another problem for schools to face, even as they undergo budget cuts, the crisis in public health becomes another problem for the police to solve. In New York, 911 emergency calls increased from 20,843 in 1980 to 46,845 in 1988.[38] Experts maintain that the release of former psychiatric patients, the growing number of homeless people and cuts in Federal funding for drug and alcohol treatment have all contributed to the increase in the police workload. Public health problems become police problems when other remedies have been eliminated by budget cuts or freezes. In some 40 percent of the cases in New York City the person whose behavior initiated the call is taken by police to a psychiatric facility.[39]

The state of New York has decreased the number of its psychiatric beds from a onetime high of 93,000 to 15,000, while another reduction of 2,000 beds is planned.[40] While their release is offered as a humanitarian solution consistent with a commitment to civil rights, many of the released individuals' health problems become a police problem. "It's a tremendous problem with a potential for people getting hurt," states Alice T. McGillion, the first deputy police commissioner. "It also requires an enormous response from the department. It has cost us a lot of time and psychic energy."[41]

It cannot be said with any sort of scientific precision that cutbacks in public health and the public health system (not that there truly was such a system even before the cutbacks in funding) directly "causes," in part, the drug crisis. The scientific precision that can justify the use of the word "cause" is the outcome of the application of mathematics to controlled experiments investigating the inorganic world. The social world and human social nature is too open-ended, too human and indeterminate for cut-and-dried mathematical formulation.

What we have instead of a demonstrable and mathematically precise "cause" is a judgement, a judgement that serves to connect a selection of facts. If for no other reason then that a selection process does occur (for the sensible reason that we cannot study everything, all at once, in all possible directions), the facts cannot be said to have been chosen without the application of this judgement. Once they have been selected, then indeed the facts may "speak for themselves." That is the substance of what an argument is. Finally, it rests on human judgement and not on "proof" as science understands it.

In regard to cutbacks in public health creating a crisis in public health, this is fairly straightforward. Following cutbacks related to public health, there occurred an increase in poverty, in hunger, and in infant mortality rates (to use three markers of social and public health). Only the latter is seriously disputed by anyone. Therefore, this issue is worth some attention.

Though data shows a marked jump in infant mortality rates in underclass neighborhoods (which were monitored), critics note that short-term statistical jumps or declines are typical and independent of variables such as funding levels. The counter argument (accepted here) is that this is merely explaining away data, for nowhere in those neighborhoods that have been measured has there been a decline in infant mortality rates. Instead, all measures show increases. If statistical flukes were at work, we should expect to find both increases and decreases in various study sites. The articles that served as the main source of the substance of the argument presented here are from *Scientific American*[42] and *Science*.[43]

In a genuine sense, the crisis in public health, along with the medicine society and other factors noted in Part One, also helps to generate the problem, particularly in underclass neighborhoods where inadequate schooling, nutrition and health care make youths (and adults) prey to drug usage and/or drug marketeering. However, as previously noted, we must always remember that the drug crisis is a classless, ethnicity-less social phenomenon. We all live in the medicine society and the medicine society crosses over all boundaries and into all neighborhoods. Given this fact, we would expect to find the worst of the crisis of usage in those neighborhoods and among those people who do not have access to drug treatment programs, and we do.

The difference between economic classes is the availability of relief. Those who have private health plans have the availability of professional experts. Those on public health plans such as Medicaid have the meager resources that public expenditures provide. Those without either (some 17 percent of the population) make do as best they can. Given that a public health system would support individual initiative and sensibility (nothing can replace that), such a system would help the whole of American society. However, in this country we have barely the embryo of a public health system, and consequently we, as a society, are prey to such crises.

The lack of a public health system exists equally with the social evils of poverty and hunger. Put together, these crises become the basis for the American problem with crime: an ever-increasing crime rate that is already the highest in the developed world. Crime is a problem that all other developed societies have solved, at least relative to The United States. The American crime rate also must be understood, in part, as a further effect of the health care delivery crisis combined with the problems of poverty and hunger.

Public health is the Achilles heel of the American system. The negative effects of the failure to make a commitment to public health show up in all sorts of statistics and facts. Were this country to make a serious effort to meet the challenge of these multiple social crises rather than search for scapegoats (always the poorest and most disenfranchised of our society), then it would make a commitment to public health.

What must be understood now is this: how is it that such a commitment has not been made? Judging from political speeches, there is no lack of commitment to either public health or the drug crisis. What happens between the speech and the action? The fact is that we are a nation that sees health as a matter of individual responsibility. The sole method of social intervention acceptable to a majority of political leaders and the public is the police. Not that this is a deliberate social policy, rather it is social policy by default.

There is the thinking that the problem is deviant individuals; therefore the response is to increase law enforcement in order that these individuals may be arrested. But such an option, given that the underlying conditions producing the problem, such as the medicine society, are beyond the scope of law enforcement, creates a self-fulfilling prophesy. And given that there is a host of problems that go along with the use of law enforcement, combined with the cutbacks in public health funding, the more law enforcement is supported, the worse the drug crisis will become.

Notes

1. Philip Caper, "Solving the Medical Care Dilemma," *New England Journal of Medicine* 318 (June 1988): 1535-36.
2. Arthur J. Barsky, "The Paradox of Health," *New England Journal of Medicine* 318 (February 1988): 414-18.
3. Ibid., 415.
4. Philip Caper, "Solving the Medical Care Dilemma," *New England Journal of Medicine* 318 (June 1988): 1535-36.
5. "Forgotten Patients," *Newsweek*, 22 August 1989, 52-53.
6. J. Larry Brown, "Hunger in the U.S.," *Scientific American*, 256 (February 1987): 39.
7. Ibid., 40.
8. Stephen Budiansky, "A Measure of Failure," *Atlantic Monthly* 257 (January 1986): 32-34.
9. Brown, "Hunger in the U.S.," 41.
10. Ibid., 40.
11. Budiansky, "A Measure of Failure," 37.
12. "Children's Health Seen As Declining," *New York Times,* 2 March 1989, I 21:1.
13. Ibid.
14. Ibid.
15. "Small Inner-City Hospitals in U.S. Face Threat of Financial Failure," *New York Times*, 21 August 1989, I 1:4.
16. Ibid., 15.
17. Ibid. Dr. Young is also a Professor of preventive medicine at the University of Illinois Medical School.
18. "Washington Talk," *New York Times*, 9 September 1988, I 10:1.
19. Ibid.
20. Ibid.
21. "Crowded County Hospitals Suffer Crisis in Obstetrics," *Los Angeles Times*, 20 February 1990, A1:1.
22. "Funds to Save Emergency Rooms Set," *Los Angeles Times*, 24 August 1988, I 1:6.
23. Ibid., I 1.
24. "Trauma in the Emergency Room," *Newsweek*, 16 February 1987, 76-77.
25. Ibid., 76.
26. Ibid.
27. Ibid.
28. "Angry Psychiatrists Denounce Threatened Mental Health Cuts," *Los Angeles Times*, 14 March 1989, I 3:1.
29. Ibid., I 3.
30. Ibid., I 20.
31. Director of the State Division of Substance Abuse Services, Julio A. Martinez, quoted in "Treating Drug Addicts: Who Should Pay For It?" *New York Times*, 27 February 1989, I 15.
32. Parole board member Ernest Salomon, quoted in "Probation Demand Tough For Addicts," *Santa Barbara News-Press*, 29 August 1989.

33. "Aid For Indigent Addicts Failing, L.A. Study Finds," *Los Angeles Times*, 1 October 1991, A 1:4.
34. "When Drugs and Despair Vie With 3R's," *New York Times*, 15 November 1989, I 1:2.
35. Ibid., I 1.
36. Ibid., II 9.
37. Ibid.
38. "Emotionally Ill Pose Growing Burden to Police," *New York Times*, 16 November 1989, A 1:2.
39. Ibid., A 1.
40. Ibid.
41. Ibid., A 19.
42. Brown, "Hunger in the U.S.," 37-41.
43. Timothy M. Smeeding and Barbara Boyld Torrey, "Poor Children in Rich Countries," *Science* 242 (November 1988): 873-77.

5

Drug Usage, Treatment, and Education

This section began by addressing the question of control, meaning, how are the would-be agents of social control, the institutions that should be alleviating the crisis, doing at their job? Social mitigators can be understood here as the equivalent of medical treatment, those systems in place that support the natural healer, individual decision-making. To the extent that there is a crisis of usage and to the extent that that crisis has been eased, the argument presented here is that individual initiative and judgement has been the prime mitigator.

However, there is a question that has yet to be addressed: just what are the problems that must be solved? In other words, what are the behavioral consequences of drug usage and how serious they? Given that the present administration has proposed spending over $10 billion on the drug problem, with state and local agencies adding another $5 billion (as a point of reference, the federal government spends $1.5 billion on public health), what is the point of such expenditures? How genuine is the problem such expenditures supposedly address?

We can understand the negative effects of drug usage to be of two sorts: social-behavioral problems associated with drug use and then, treated separately because of its prominence in public debate, the problem of crime. These can be understood as the primary, direct effects of drug use. Nonetheless, it should be noted that there are alternative understandings of drugs. Aldous Huxley, for example, noted that "...people were pharmacologists before they were farmers."[1] Moreover, there is a long history of individuals across time and across cultures using alcohol/drugs in their social celebrations.

We should also know something about the effectiveness of drug treatment. Given the argument that the primary motivation is individual judgement, it follows that social policy should be directed toward strengthening individual judgement. This means, in part, drug treatment and drug education programs. Certainly, the reader must anticipate that increased expenditures for drug treatment clinics will be part of the eventual proposed policy. We should know if such treatment does any good. Then, making the common sense assumption it must do some good, the question becomes: how much good? Furthermore, drug education is often called for; what does the research show regarding the effectiveness of such education? First, the issue of effects will be considered, and then the research reports about the links between drugs and crime will be examined. Last, reports about drug treatment and drug education will be presented.

Before moving on to statistical reports, the first consideration must be that the alcohol/drug effects to be reported on occur in a particular sort of culture with particular sorts of generalized customs and attitudes toward alcohol and drug usage. In other words, the "objective" facts are embedded within a particular culture and we must understand that this particular culture, a culture composed of individuals with these generalized notions of how and when and what is appropriate to consume, is producing these figures and not the "drugs" themselves.

What might this mean? For example, alcohol can be considered a "dangerous" drug, a drug responsible for 100,000 deaths a year, as well as $120 billion a year in economic losses and a drug highly correlated with violence and abusive behavior toward children. These facts are true but, nonetheless, it would be wrong to thereby conclude that a "drug," per se, is producing these statistics. How so?

Jewish-Americans consume just about as much alcohol as any ethnic group. Indeed, they consume more than most American ethnic groups. However, the Jewish alcoholic is rare and all the problems statistically associated with alcohol use are quite infrequent among Jewish-Americans. In other words, even as we should know the behaviors correlated with alcohol use when considering problematic behaviors and alcohol/drug usage, we should never erase the human and cultural factors. People are powerful, not drugs, and it is a people, not a drug, that is producing the statistics.

Researchers point out that alcohol use among Jewish people is ritualized, done at the dinner table (while eating, the eating itself buffering the alcohol) with family (done openly rather than covertly), and celebrated as a part of the living of their religion (rather than as a somewhat disrespectable behavior). At the same time, alcohol is not used to become intoxicated; alcohol use is fully and explicitly social, part of the gathering together of family and friends.

Moreover, the Jewish people, while openly enjoying their social drink, on the other hand severely condemn and openly disapprove of drunkenness. In other words, quoting Charles R. Snyder, the Jewish people have "...ritualized the use of beverage alcohol; he has brought drinking within the sphere of the most powerful social controls and moral sentiments."[2]

This cultural context is far removed from the usual American drinking context. In the usual American home, drinking is not done at the dinner table with family—instead one goes out to a dimly lit bar to perform the disrespectable behavior. Furthermore, being "drunk" is thought understandable, humorous, even desirable—not stigmatizing—for it is the very purpose of drinking. The apparent purpose of drinking is to achieve disrespectability. Hence, the act itself is somewhat disrespectable (thus not done at home but away) and the achievement of drunkenness is understood as the successful culmination of the disrespectable act. In other words, if a culture that preferred alcohol wanted to maximize the harm the use of the drug might bring, that culture would be sure to imbue drinking with much if not all of the attitudes typical of our own.

With the cultural context of alcohol/drug usage in mind, the following summarizes the research upon behavior and alcohol/drug use.

What Are the Social-Behavioral Effects of Drug Usage?

There are any number of studies on the connection between drug usage and problematic behavior. A critical question is the problem of causality: in cases of problematic drug usage and problematic behavior, which is the real "cause"? Does some sort of psychopathology lead to the problematic usage, or did the problematic usage come first and create the social/behavioral difficulty? Examples of both sorts of arguments can be found in the literature.

The argument is also raised that addictions, particularly alcoholism, are genetic-based, that an "alcoholic" gene is passed on from father to son. Curiously, such proponents do not make the same argument for female alcoholism. This argument received much attention in the press and is thereby worth extended consideration following this introduction.

Then there is a fourth line of reasoning—that some third variable, psychological rather than physiological, preceded and "caused" both the problematic usage and the problematic behavior. There is a fifth angle as well: that we can best understand instances of chronic usage and problematic behavior as an unfolding process in which drug usage and psychopathology interact to maintain the continued presence of each. Below, representative examples will be given of each sort of interpretation.

An example of the first model of causality, drug usage creating the psychopathology, comes from a research report by Marc Schuckit.[3] Schuckit notes that symptoms of depression are very common in alcoholics. This creates a clinical problem: which is the symptom and which is the underlying condition, the alcoholism or the depression? The typical inpatient treatment is to detoxify the patient first and, if the depression continues, then it is treated. Generally though, the depression lifts following detoxification. Presumably, the same sort of thinking is followed in drug treatment as well.

Examples of the second sort of explanation, psychopathology generating problematic drug usage, can be found in the literature on children of alcoholics. Researchers note that a person from an alcoholic family is three to four times more likely to become an alcoholic than a person from a non-alcoholic family. Joan Jackson is generally credited with being the therapist/researcher who introduced the notion of the "alcoholic family."[4] Present-day writing describes such a family as being in denial of the presence of alcoholism in a family member; in denial of how family relationships have crystallized around the problem; and finally, in denial of themselves. Following Claudia Black's work, this is often put as "don't think, don't feel, don't trust" sort of thinking.[5]

The "denial/survivor" model then describes siblings whose successful adaptation to a difficult social situation at home renders the same person maladjusted outside the home. In other words, having adjusted to unhealthy relationships, the person cannot form healthy relationships. Moreover, the person is described as one whose psychological adjustments, made to endure the home situation, include a denial of self and a tendency to compulsive behaviors that can make self-growth highly unlikely.[6]

It is an open question if this model could be brought to bear on the understanding of the "drug family." The presumption here is that the use of a different drug would not plausibly change the nature of the family's problem. In addition to the "alcoholic family," the dysfunctional family is said to socialize the offspring into compulsive behaviors, including alcohol and substance abuse. This is an example of the second sort of causal pathway, a psychopathology creating the addiction.

There are those who maintain that "genetics" can account for the higher prevalence. However, any argument that puts "genetics" forward as a cause for problematic behavior rests not upon a precise understanding of how "genetics" affect behavior, but rather, any such argument rests upon researcher's and practitioner's fundamental ignorance of how genetics might produce behaviors. Hence, any such argument based upon a found correlation (such as between having an alcoholic father and being an alcoholic), rests upon our ignorance of genetics and behavior: in other words, our inability to demonstrate or to explain the existence of a genuine or spurious correlation.

Contrary evidence is found in a 17 year study of 420 families. Researchers here found that the offspring of heavy drinkers were just as likely to be abstainers or light drinkers as heavy drinkers, and that most heavy drinkers came from families of moderate drinking parents. But there were all sorts of variations given the gender of the heavy drinking parent and the gender of the offspring. The greatest probability of finding a heavy drinking offspring occurred when both parents were heavy drinkers.

Nonetheless, the critical problem of explanation remains—finding a theory that explains the exceptions as well as the rule. Given the inability of any one theory to do this, neither psychological- nor physiological-based explanations can be dismissed out of hand. Social psychological factors may explain most alcoholism and abuse and genetics the cases of extreme abuse and disinterest in recovery.

The psychological theory remains useful given its flexibility and applicability—but at the expense of any precision. The genetic theory is precise but unprovable and irrefutable—again, given our ignorance of how a defective gene (not yet found) produces alcohol abuse (itself better defined by common sense than by science).

One more point before returning to the next causal explanation of alcohol/drug abuse: the Federal government has swallowed the genetic argument hook, line, and sinker. The *Sixth Annual Report to Congress on Alcohol Health* (1987) by the National Institute of Alcoholism and Alcohol Abuse states *all* male alcoholism is generated by genetics, with social and psychological factors given one sentence of attention.[7] The political benefits of the genetic argument, quite unintended by researchers, is that if alcohol/drug abuse is created by "bad genes," then there is no need for fundamental political and social change to deal with the drug crisis. This is probably why the government so favors it. Nonetheless, the research into genetics and addiction remains intriguing and well worth the research effort.

Another general interpretation of alcohol/drug abuse is of some third psychological factor, something other than the drug use or the problematic behavior itself, that is proposed to generate both. For example, in one study of a sample of women who had reported a sexual dysfunction of some sort, the women were divided into two matched groups on the basis of being an alcoholic or not. The study ("Women, Alcohol and Sexuality") was undertaken by Stephanie S. Covington and Janet Kohen and reported in 1984. They found that "alcoholic women experienced more sexual abuse, of a more extreme nature, and were more likely to experience the abuse over a longer period of their lives."[8]

Further, the alcoholic women were more likely to have suffered chronic physical abuse. Thus the finding was that the suffering of sexual and/or physical abuse while young makes it more likely that a woman will become alcoholic and will report sexual dysfunctions. Nonetheless, many of the individuals who reported sexual or physical abuse when young were *not* alcoholic. Statements of populations cannot be directly translated into statements about individuals. What is true of individuals is endless variation.

Then there is a fifth kind of causal interpretation, of problematic drug usage and problematic behavior interacting and continuing together. A specific example of this comes from a study by Herbert Hending and Ann Pollinger of chronic marijuana use reported in 1985. The study, which included and compared adult usage with adolescent usage, found of adolescent heavy marijuana users: "In all of its functions, marijuana served to detach these adolescents from the problems of the real world—from their anger and unhappiness with their parents, and from the need to work and compete to achieve success."[9] The reporters further stressed that they were not stating that marijuana use preceded personal problems nor the reverse. Rather, heavy marijuana use was an adaptive response, a "...characteristic, definable, defensive role in these students' attempts to deal with conflict over competition and aggression which had become intolerable."[10]

Two difficulties with this study are the low number of research subjects (only 17) and the problem of normative bias. For example, adolescents who used marijuana were said to argue with their parents and this was explained as an example of problematic behavior associated with chronic marijuana usage. The difficulty, of course, is sorting through the usual parent/adolescent conflicts and those (if any) distinct to marijuana users. In addition, "chronic" usage is an apparently meaningful term but really is not. For example, weekly use of cocaine is considered problematic or chronic, but if the same measure was to be applied to alcohol, some 70 percent of the population would be found to be "chronic" drinkers. Nonetheless, reporting the researcher's interpretation, chronic drug usage and problematic behavior are intertwined, each reinforcing the other. Moreover, this is consistent with the general understanding of the field.[11]

So there are five different types of causal explanations for alcohol/drug use and problematic behavior that can be found in the literature. Which one is right? The difficulty in answering such a question is that none have proven to be of significant usefulness in the treatment of problematic drug usage. Moreover, the validity of such theories cannot be based upon the facts alone for, by definition, such causal theories seek to go beyond the facts to "explain" the "facts." The bottom line is that no practitioner or researcher can demonstrate how their explanation is the superior one in either the general or the specific case.

Apparently, practitioners and researchers are apt to perceive or be interested in those factors that they have been trained to perceive, with no one perception demonstrably superior to another. Of course, it is not just a matter of perception; the problem is multidimensional and complex. As Thomas McCellan of the Philadelphia Veteran's Administration Hospital is quoted: "Almost anything you state about alcoholics is bound to be true of some, but nothing is going to be true for all."[12]

Therefore, it appears better to sidestep the issues of "cause" and interpretations of pathology and proceed to the overt problematic behaviors associated with the most common drugs. Given the boundaries of our knowledge of physiology and psychology, "cause" is bound to be a problematic word. However, we can specify the problems associated with drug usage in a definitive way and this will prove more useful than speculations upon "cause." There is a social universe of unique individuals; nonetheless, regularities emerge in studies of populations. The following report summarizes those regularities.

The most replicated findings in the field of alcohol and drug abuse relevant to the social-behavioral effects of drugs are the high correlations between alcohol use and divorce, spouse abuse, child abuse, and child sexual abuse. In other words, there is not just a general sort of pathology found in drug usage; in the case of alcohol, there are specific behavioral problems. Moreover, these problems can be extreme and have extraordinary consequences for the children who suffer at the hands of alcoholic parents.

However, this is not to say that all alcoholic parents abuse their children or spouses. As is often true, the specific facts can be paradoxical. For example, one report shows that heavy drinking parent(s) will avoid their children specifically to minimize the potential of harming them.[13] Still, as will be noted, one of the most replicated of findings is the correlation between alcohol use and aggression of all sorts.

In addition to the correlations between alcohol use and domestic violence, there are high correlations of alcohol use and psychopathology of all sorts, in particular depression and suicide. Alcohol abuse is also highly correlated with physical illnesses of all kinds. In a study performed at Johns Hopkins University, 13 percent to 30 percent (depending upon the particular medical department) of patients admitted to the hospital were found to be alcoholics.[14] All of these patients were admitted under diagnoses other than alcoholism.

Alcohol use is also highly correlated with self-injury such as: death by falling (48 percent of those dying by falls were legally intoxicated or had alcohol in their bloodstream), by fire (54 percent), and by drowning (53 percent) according to one study.[15] Of course, alcohol use is highly correlated with traffic fatalities. The National Institute of Justice estimates between 5 percent and 10 percent of all weekend drivers are under the influence and that alcohol is a factor in some 60 percent of all traffic fatalities and in some 90 percent of all traffic accidents. In all, the *Journal of the American Medical Association* estimates that the effects of alcohol costs the country some $120 billion a year.[16]

It is possible these problems are linked to alcohol because of the wide availability of this particular drug and were other drugs equally available we would find the same problems and to the same degree. The one difficulty with this assumption is that illegal drugs are virtually as available as alcohol. Second, though usage rates of the most widely used illegal drug, marijuana, is approximately one-third that of alcohol, this drug does not show up as co-existing with the problems of assault, child abuse, suicide, self-injury, or any of the other problems noted above. Cocaine, however, is beginning to show up in some of the same kinds of statistics formerly associated only with alcohol.

In a recent study, cocaine was found in the bloodstream of one-quarter of the individuals who died in car accidents. And, in a somewhat misleading study, of all Los Angeles coroner's cases found positive for the presence of drugs, 60 percent had died a violent death. (This is misleading given the county's rather large gang problem and, furthermore, limiting the report to only those cases that included the presence of drugs is bound to exaggerate the results.) Nonetheless, this is an indication that at least some of the social/behavioral effects of cocaine may be quite similar to alcohol, and that increasing use of cocaine will lead to increasing amounts of some of the same sorts of problems related to alcohol use. These two drugs (along with heroin) also figure prominently in the section on drugs and crime.

From this author's unpublished and preliminary research, there are further statements that can be made with regard to cocaine and alcohol: individuals responsible for the care and protection of infants born with drugs in their bloodstream have reported that alcoholic or cocaine-abusing parent(s) appear to be the most irresponsible and uncaring of parents. A doctor responsible for the care of such infants noted that cocaine-abusing parent(s) often appear uncaring about even naming a child and are often unconcerned about leaving the hospital without the child. Furthermore, a person responsible for the protection of such infants stated that even heroin-addicted mothers and fathers are more concerned over their children than either cocaine or alcohol abusing-parents.[17]

We have touched briefly on the effects of chronic or dangerous use; what are the effects of occasional drug use?

An eight-year study tracked adolescent drug use and its impact in some 739 Los Angeles area youths.[18] As a population (rather than as individuals, since what is true of individuals is unpredictable variation), casual use of drugs was found to have no significant physical health risk. The health scores of the population of casual users equalled the health scores of non-users. However, there was a direct and linear relationship between amounts of drug usage and psychological problems: the greater the drug use, the greater the problems. The researchers also found that heavy drug use affected nearly every dimension of social and behavioral health.

The UCLA study noted: "The typical youngster who has a beer or some marijuana at a party is not the one who is going to develop long-term damage as a result of their drug use," according to the researchers. "It is those teenagers who develop a life style of drug use to relieve emotional distress and other life stressors...that will suffer long-term, negative consequences of their use."[19]

But such an outcome was not popular with either politicians or parents. The National Institute of Drug Abuse (NIDA) reported dozens of queries about the study and, according to one report, parents (and the White House) were furious that such an outcome was reported. "Drug use is a very emotional issue," Robert J. Pandina, a Rutgers University psychologist working on a similar project is quoted in response to the reaction to the study. He then adds: "When you provide an unpopular message in a political process, you're likely to get hammered for it."[20]

Nonetheless, Pandina's own study of 1,400 New Jersey youths followed for more than a decade appears to be replicating the UCLA study. "In many studies, the findings, I think, are fairly consistent," Pandina reports in a Los Angeles Times interview appearing in August 1988. "While there may be occasional problems, those problems are really episodic. They are not of the same nature as those of chronic drug users."[21] He goes on to note: "Not that it's not risky behavior. But there's a lot of risky behavior. It's not the rapid, escalating use leading to heroin abuse. We're just not finding that."[22]

Such findings may be controversial when linked with the illegal drugs but find ready acceptance when linked with alcohol. For example, the National Institute of Justice, in a release on the effects of alcohol consumption, closed the release with the caveat that, despite the many and severe problematic effects of alcohol consumption, nonetheless, there are "...tens of millions of people who find alcohol consumption a major pleasure in life and who themselves drink responsibly."[23] No such caveat in any context is found when the subject is some other drug.

One more study on drug effects is useful to quote here. John D. Hundleby ("Drug Usage and Outstanding Performance Among Young Adolescents") studied the school performances of some 2,000 ninth grade boys and girls. The correlations between outstanding performance in school and drug usage were small but significant. However, the best predictor of not being an outstanding performer was the use of a drug not usually associated with problem behavior: tobacco.[24]

How might all such research be generalized and in such a way as to include drugs not examined, for example, psychedelics? The following is proposed: generally put, alcohol/drug usage runs the risk of various sorts of physical ailments, dependency, and avoidance behavior. Even marijuana, the drug least associated with physical ailments, creates the problem of lung damage. Further, given that drugs are taken to produce positive effects, there is the danger of learning to become dependent upon those effects. Competition and conflict are inevitable facts of life. Alcohol/drug usage can provide a handy, if false, exit from facing the challenge of that competition and conflict. Moreover, there are specific dangers associated with specific drugs, for example, alcohol use and aggressive behavior. In addition, the drug least associated with behavioral changes is physiologically the most dangerous of drugs, tobacco.

Drugs and Crime

One of the oldest and most replicated findings in studies of drugs and crime is the high correlation between alcohol and assaultive behavior; in more than one-half of homicides, assaults and rapes, the perpetrator had been drinking. Furthermore, as acts of aggression become more violent, the likelihood that the aggressor has consumed alcohol prior to the assault increases dramatically.

Another facet of alcohol usage is the high correlation between using alcohol and being a victim of a crime. For example, in a study of homicide victims in Erie County, New York, and in Los Angeles, some 60 percent of all victims were found to have alcohol in their bloodstream. There are a number of such studies that find approximately the same percentage and this holds true for other violent crimes, such as assault and rape. The usual explanation given is that the consumption of alcohol leads people to perform unsafe behaviors, such as leaving friends behind, going into unsafe areas or simply being out alone at night while obviously vulnerable, acts that the individuals probably would not have performed had they been sober.

There is evidence now that illicit drugs of all kinds are also becoming as commonplace a correlation as alcohol in the commission of crime. One study of 2,000 individuals arrested for property or violent crime found that some 50 to 75 percent of such individuals had illegal drugs in their bloodstream. Though the study is flawed in that possession of drugs was included in the count, still, according to the National Institute of Justice, this was the exception rather than the rule for the population that was sampled.[25]

Perhaps predictably, this evidence leads one group of interpreters (primarily from the Justice Department) to conclude that more money needs to be spent on the law enforcement option, while another group, primarily non-government experts, conclude that this makes the case for more drug treatment programs.

What is probably happening is nothing remarkable at all. Given the historically high correlations between alcohol and violent crime, and the present high (relatively) usage rates of illicit drugs, it makes sense that any number of individuals are going to be substituting an illegal drug for the legal drug of alcohol. The connection between drug use and crime is as problematic as the connection between drug use and psychopathology. Indeed, that crime, particularly violent crime, is not considered evidence of psychopathology is a social definition only, it is hard to find the difference in the act itself.

A fourth critical finding of drugs and crime (besides alcohol and assaultive behavior, alcohol use and being a victim of a crime, and the emerging reports of similar correlations with cocaine) is the often verified correlation between heroin usage and property crime. The National Institute of Justice reports astonishing rates of commission of property crime correlated with heroin usage. According to one report, daily heroin users were found to commit on average some 300 non-drug related crimes a year, primarily burglary, theft and shoplifting.

More critically and more interestingly, the problem of drugs and crime is primarily an underclass problem. This is the fifth critical correlation of drugs, and crime. This is not to be expected if the naive explanation is accepted, that the use of drugs turns individuals, in some mysterious way, into dangerous criminals. Middle- and higher-income individuals consume illicit drugs but such usage in these classes is not associated with criminal activity (beyond the drug activity itself). The high correlation of drug use and crime is only true of the underclass. This indicates that something other than the naive explanation of the connection between drugs and crime is happening. What might this be?

The first part of the explanation has already been given: the connection between drugs and crime, in the absence of sophisticated drug treatment programs, becomes a self-fulfilling prophesy. Lacking treatment possibilities, it appears inevitable that the alternative, the police station, will be required, at least for many of the underclass with problematic drug usage.

Moreover, the correlation found between drugs and crime and the underclass is but another manifestation of the general malaise of this class. The failure to mitigate the pathology producing the conditions of this class (such as lack of health care and endemic malnutrition), generates all sorts of statistics: infant mortality, crime rates, problematic drug usage—virtually any sort of social statistic that might be mentioned. Initially, these problems are the problems of the underclass, but they become problems for the rest of society as, for example, when gang violence breaks out of underclass neighborhoods and invades middle-class neighborhoods.

Though the naive connection between drugs and crime was much pushed by the Reagan administration, the Bush administration appears to be backing away from this argument. Current drug czar Bob Martinez, for example, is quoted as rejecting the naive explanation and further stating: "There are other social pathologies at work which will continue to foster violence, especially in our cities."[26] The next question of relevance here becomes how much of a real alternative is drug treatment and drug education? According to the research, how well do they work?

Drug Treatment

There are some 43 distinct theories of the causes of addiction and dependency. They all make good sense and one of them just might be right. The difficulty in sorting them out is that no approach to addiction can be found that is clearly superior to another. When cure rates are examined, no one approach has been found that works particularly better than another, or even particularly well at all. This can be compared to the medical sciences, in which the success of disease theory (meaning, find the pathogen creating the problem, destroy the pathogen, and the disease is thereby cured) has created a unified field of understanding and treatment of physical ills. The treatment of psychological ills has yet to find that successful principle around which research and practice can crystallize. Hence, there is a plethora of theory combined with a paucity of successful results.

But again, any work with the addicted means working with the most difficult of populations—-individuals who have found themselves unable to exercise individual sensibility and judgement and who have a problem that can only be resolved by the exercise of such. This is the dilemma of drug treatment and why treatment is so tenuous. Even as medical science is disarmed and disabled in the absence of the body's natural healers, so too are the psychological sciences.

There are specific findings in the research on drug treatment:

(1) There is a critical gender variable. Women, even as they consistently show lower usage rates, also show higher rates of successful treatment. According to a 1985 study by Fred Holsten ("The Female Drug Abuser: Has She a Shorter Way Out?"): "The way out of drug abuse took less time for females than for males...[and] females had a better prognosis than males after both a short and longer observation periods."[27]

The critical conclusions were: "Compared to males, females are less involved with criminality, often have lighter abuse, and often are more occupied with their relationships with other partners."[28] Indeed, this concern with relationships was proposed as the means by which the female abuser finds her way out of her drug abuse.

There are also critical gender differences in usage. Generally, women show lower rates of drug usage and abuse than men. However, there is one sort of drug women, particularly younger women, are more likely to abuse than men—stimulants. Presumably, this use is related to weight control. Second, women are more likely than men to have a prescription for tranquilizers, anti-depressants or sedative-hypnotics.

(2) Alcohol, heroin, and tobacco are considered by many researchers to be the most addictive of all drugs. Dependent users of any of these three drugs show nearly identical relapse rates following treatment. About two-thirds of all relapses occur within the first ninety days following treatment for any of these three drugs. By twelve months, 80 percent of heroin users and tobacco users have suffered relapse and about 70 percent of alcohol users. This data is from a standard work in the field edited by G. Alan Marlatt, *Relapse Prevention*. Simply put, in the case of these drugs, relapse is predictable. Everett Koop, former Surgeon-General of the Reagan

administration, has also equaled nicotine addiction with heroin addiction.[29]

Nonetheless, many researchers caution against painting any simple picture of treatment outcomes. Vaillant, in *The Natural History of Alcoholism*, produced an oft-referred-to work that summarizes and analyzes the critical studies of alcoholism. He notes that long-term studies find many alcoholics achieving limited periods of abstinence, or at least non-problematic drinking. Such facts complicate considerably any reports on treatment outcomes. It becomes critical *when* the alcoholic or recovered alcoholic was counted in the research, when they were "on the wagon" or off. This refers to research on relapse rates.

Furthermore, Vaillant noted that many reports do not account for alcoholics who have died in the course of the study nor do studies control for a standard fact of alcoholism and the alcoholic, the premature death rate long associated with this group. This makes a difference when reporting the numbers of drinkers who have either given up drinking or given up trying to. The latter figure in particular will be exaggerated if drinkers who died are not discounted.

The general truth appears to be that for most alcoholics, the alcoholism develops over the course of a 10 to 15 year period and their alcoholism is going to be a persistent feature of their life. Treatments will be effective for a time, but periods of abstinence will alternate with bouts of drinking. The general truth will be that their alcohol addiction is a lifetime struggle.

Regarding cocaine, this drug is apparently more amenable to treatment than alcohol, heroin, or tobacco, at least according to a number of preliminary reports. This makes sense when one considers that cocaine does not appear to produce a physiological dependency (as do the other three drugs). However, another possibility is that this drug has been less extensively researched than the others; hence, early reports about the effectiveness of treatment could be more optimistic than is warranted.

(3) There are a number of findings on the correlation of the type of treatment given and the outcome of the treatment. Pulling together all of the reports eventually results in more ambiguity than clarity. However, given the reason for ambiguity and the prominence of the alternative of drug treatment in the current debate, it is worthwhile to consider this aspect.

First, there is no recommended single method for drug treatment: the treatment of addiction is thought to be most effective when a combination of approaches are used, including drug therapy, psychotherapy, and group therapy. Drug therapy is thought to hold the best hope for an eventual "cure," perhaps paradoxically—but then this is the medicine society and drugs do cure.[30]

Additionally, for the mild-to-moderately addicted (which is not to say that drug/alcohol therapists would agree there is such a person), a study published in the *New England Journal of Medicine* by Dr. Motoi Hayashida and colleagues found that outpatient detoxification and treatment worked as well as inpatient treatment.[31]

What does make a difference in treatment outcomes? From a study of 1,091 alcoholics in a variety of treatment services, followed for one year, the finding was that group therapy proved more effective than individual therapy. In addition, there was the finding that the longer the duration of treatment, the lower the relapse rates.

However, these intuitively sensible findings are questioned by at least one review of the literature, which found no significant differences in outcome given varying lengths of stay and intensity of treatment.[32] Here, we are faced once more with the problem of applying science to individual and social behavior—one finds similar and opposite answers. Why? The great confounding variable is people.

Inanimate matter is regular and predictable, people are not. Not only are there all sorts of responses to treatment, there are all sorts of treatments applied with varying levels of skills. Further, the most critical factor, the determination of the abuser to change, is the most immeasurable. So the correlation between type of treatment and success rate is ambiguous. However, more solid ground can be found when the question is posed thus: are there social and psychological factors in regard the client that are useful in predicting success?

(4) The fourth critical fact of treatment comes from a study performed by Reginald G. Smart. This researcher found that the characteristics of patients are more important in predicting successful treatment than the type of treatment received. Whether employed or not, degrees of social stability (measured by such variables as finances, employment stability, and lack of legal problems, among others), life conditions (a person's satisfaction with his or her life and relationships with the significant others), all proved more critical than the type of treatment in predicting the outcome of treatment.[33] In addition, personality characteristics may matter: alcoholics who do not abuse other drugs, or alcoholics who are

prone to depression as opposed to anti-social behavior are reported to do better in treatment.

Much of this is immediately relevant to the underclass problem within the drug crisis. Such individuals discover drug treatment of any kind is hard to find. In New York, for example, it is estimated that in 1983 there were 97,000 crack users under the age of 16, but there were only 150 beds for inpatient treatment. For the state there are 10,000 outpatient treatment slots, but this is a total and these youngsters are competing with all drug treatment seekers for these slots.

But, if the research reports upon the impact of the person's immediate social environment are correct, then the problem is larger than drug treatment per se. The very conditions necessary for recovery are the same conditions absent in the lives of many underclass youths. Once again, the problem is a general lack of health and care. The question becomes: what is the consequence of not addressing this need and of substituting law enforcement for public health?

The law enforcement option: the police station as the emergency room and then jail as the ineffectual and backward hospital of American social ills, this becomes the solution. In this way, the equation of drugs with crime becomes a self-fulfilling prophesy. Lacking treatment facilities for underclass youth, and given the need for sophisticated treatment for the cure of addiction and dependency, as well as a supportive environment for recovery, people without the availability of such cures, or at least a large number of them, are bound to end up in the back of police cruisers. Present policy inevitably produces such results.

One more note regarding the availability of drug treatment: it is not just the uninsured that find such treatment scarce; so do mothers-to-be. Clinics would rather not treat pregnant women because of potential liability problems. Hence, according to an account given by one expert, mothers-to-be are another group that finds this sort of health care beyond their reach—even if they are insured.[34]

Regarding the effectiveness of alcohol/drug treatment in the general population, it should be noted that these reports focused upon complete cures. What was unacknowledged is that drug treatment, even when not producing total cures may, nonetheless, minimize the harm the addict/alcoholic (or problematic user) causes others. In other words, the level of the problem may be reduced by drug treatment, even if the problem is not completely "cured."

Drug Education

The Gallup Poll in March 1988 reported that 47 percent of Americans interviewed felt that drug education would do the most good in halting the drug "epidemic."[35] This was the most frequently given reply. Curiously, the younger a person was, the more likely they were to give this response, but all categories were fairly consistent.

The government disagrees. Former drug czar William Bennett, in testimony before the Senate, stated he thought drug education would do little good in preventing drug abuse among the young.[36] The budget he proposed reflected his opinion, with law enforcement receiving many times the amount of funding that drug education efforts received. What is the evidence of the effectiveness of drug education?

In June 1989, the *Journal of the American Medical Association* reported the outcome of a Kansas City metropolitan area drug education program aimed at sixth and seventh graders.[37] The drug education program included school workshops and homework assignments and local newspaper and television collaboration. The results were very encouraging. Analyses of 42 schools showed significantly lower usage rates of marijuana, tobacco, and alcohol than in the control group.[38]

The report reviewed previous findings on the effectiveness of drug education. According to this report, the critical variable determining the success of such programs is peer participation. Young people must be involved in the design and implementation of such programs if such programs are to show success. Furthermore, this age group (sixth and seventh graders) is critical; these are the years when drug experimentation begins. The researchers noted that "...more than 20 of these [recent] studies have shown significant reductions, between 29 percent and 67 percent in experimental smoking rates among adolescents, with more moderate reductions in alcohol and marijuana use."[39]

However, the researchers were also careful to note that there are contradictory reports. There is also research that indicates positive outcomes can be "...minimal to moderate and, in some cases, short-lived or delayed."[40] The usual explanation is that larger environmental factors, such as media depictions in advertisements and programming of the positive benefits of drug use, undermine the effectiveness of school-based drug education programs.Further, there is the problem of the limited scope of many school programs, "limited" referring to the number of area schools involved in the program. The outstanding feature of the Kansas City project was that all schools in the area were involved and the media was enlisted in the drug education efforts.

Nonetheless, there is research consistent with Mr. Bennett's opinion. A 1986 survey of seven different school-based education programs found them to be minimally and only briefly effective.[41] The fact is, "drug education" is no simple or straightforward thing, nor even the same thing (programs vary), nor do such programs mean the same thing to different people. Richard Blum, the author and editor of a 1976 work about education notes: "It's easy to go wrong with drug education."[42]

He points out that such education misses truants, that schools are already burdened with multiple outside objectives quite beyond the basic task of educating children in the fundamental intellectual skills, that children refer to their own experience and opinion of peers, and, as always "...what we thought we were doing and saying in the classroom seems not to be what the students perceived."[45] Apparently, what was said to discourage became a stimulus to try. Last, there is the endless variation of teaching style and content. In a sentence, there are lots of ways to go wrong in drug education and no certain way of succeeding with all young people.

There is another consideration that justifies, in part, the former drug czar's skepticism—the media can undo the effects of drug education. However, this should not mean that drug education should be abandoned, especially given the solid evidence that it works. Instead, the worst of the media influences, its never ending promotion of drug usage (drug education of the reverse sort), should become the object of change.

The advertising expenditures of behavioral drug companies will be briefly noted here (briefly, for it is covered in other sections as well). For example, the tobacco industry spends some $2.5 billion a year in advertisements. This is far more than the amount the federal government spends on drug education. Further, Surgeon General Antonia Novello has accused cigarette manufacturers of directing their promotions at children and adolescents.[44] Such promotions are undertaken by cigarette companies despite the fact that cigarette smoking was responsible for the deaths of some 390,000 individuals in 1988, and that smoking is as addictive as heroin.

Drug advertisements are only one of the ways the media promotes drug use (in other words, educates the young in the supposed positive effects of drug usage). In a study that looked at how prime-time programming depicts drug usage, alcohol usage was found to be depicted neutrally 85 percent of the time, positively 9 percent of the time and negatively 6 percent of the time.[45]

A "neutral" presentation means that individuals were shown drinking without consequence, such as impaired judgement or speech, loss of balance and so on. When alcohol use was depicted negatively, generally, this was when lower-income groups were shown drinking. When upper-income groups were shown over-drinking, it was presented as humorous and inconsequential. Alcohol use was positively associated with celebrations and romantic encounters.[46]

Despite the media's collaboration with alcohol manufacturers in the promotion of this drug, there remains the report of a decrease in drug usage following school-based drug education programs. This indicates that such programs, properly organized, are worth funding. A further point is that there is drug education going on, but it is being performed by tobacco and liquor promoters. Their message is to encourage young people to take up the use of these drugs even though, for young people, it is as illegal to purchase alcohol as it is to purchase marijuana. Following the ban on ciga-rette advertisements on television, there was a remarkable decline in the numbers of people smoking. There is every reason to believe that the same sort of decline would follow the banning of liquor promotion on television.

Three sub-themes regarding solutions to the drug problem are that alcohol and tobacco comprise a major portion of the drug cri-sis yet precious little Federal action is being taken to discourage their usage; that drug treatment and drug education are critical needs yet the current Federal budget overlooks both in favor of law-enforcement; and that the equating of drugs with crime becomes a self-fulfilling prophesy when drug treatment as well as general health care are short-changed.

Does the expense of the solution match the problem? Unlike eco-nomic crisis, social crisis defies objective measure and evaluation. If drug use was half what it is today, some would still maintain that a crisis existed and any number of politicians and bureaucrats could be found to agree. Moreover, that is exactly what has hap-pened. Usage has not halved, but usage levels (as noted elsewhere) have declined to nearly 1973 levels yet still the Washington drum-beat, dutifully echoed by the press, is heard against the usage of illegal drugs, even as the legal and more lethal drugs are diligently protected.

Still, beyond the normative nature of the use of the word "crisis," given the correlations of, for example, alcohol and aggression, spending $10 billion a year could be justified. But such spending can only be justified for drug treatment and education that includes the legal drugs (combined with legislation that would minimize the pro-drug education of alcohol advertisements), as well as for other aspects of the more general social crisis of health. Failing such expenditures, the otherwise spurious correlation of drugs and crime becomes a genuine correlation.

Notes

1. Aldous Huxley, *The Doors of Perception* (New York: Harper & Row, 1954).
2. Charles B. Snyder, *Alcohol and the Jews* (Glencoe: The Free Press, 1958). For writings on the problem of causality and drug usage, refer to John K. Watters, Craig Reinarman, and Jeffrey Fagan, "Causality, Context and Contingency: Relationships Between Drug Abuse and Delinquency," *Contemporary Drug Problems* 12 (Fall 1985): 351-73 and Milton F. Shore, "Correlates and Concepts: Are We Chasing Our Tails?" *Etiology of Drug Abuse*, Research Monograph No. 56 (Washington, DC: National Institute of Drug Abuse, 1985).
3. Marc A. Schuckit, "Alcoholism and Affective Disorders: Diagnostic Confusion," *Alcohol and Dependency*, Ed. D. W. Goodwin, (New York: Spectrum, 1984).
4. Joan Jackson, "The Adjustment of the Family to the Crisis of Alcoholism," *Quarterly Journal of Studies of Alcoholism* 15 (1954): 562-86.
5. Claudia Black, *It Will Never Happen To Me* (Denver: M.A.C., 1981).
6. There are many works out that mention this theory; Stephanie Brown, *Treating Adult Children of Alcoholics* (New York: Wiley, 1988) was the source used here. For other literature on this topic, standard sources are Claudia Black, *It Will Never Happen To Me* (Denver: M.A.C., 1981); Herbert Gravitz and Julie Bowden, *Theraputic Issues of Adult Children of Alcoholics* (Holmes Beach, FL: Learning Publications, 1985); Timmen Cermak, *Primer for Adult Children of Alcoholics* (Pompano Beach: Health Communications, 1985) and others.
7. National Institute of Alcohol Abuse and Alcoholism (NIAAA), *Sixth Annual Report to the U.S. Congress on Alcohol and Health*, DHHS Pub. No. (ADM), 97-1519 (Washington, DC: U.S. Government Printing Office). This report reduces all alcoholism to a problem of genetics.
8. Stephanie S. Covington and Janet Kohen, "Women, Alcohol and Sexuality," *Advances in Alcohol and Substance Abuse* 4 (Fall 1984): 41-56.
9. Herbert Hendin and Ann Pollinger Haas, "The Adaptive Significance of Chronic Marijuana Use for Adolescents and Adults," *Advances in Alcohol and Drug Abuse* 4 (Spring/Summer 1985): 99-115.

10. Ibid., 100.
11. For example, in a recent treatment report issued by the NIDA, the conclusion is, "...there are no simplistic predictors of drug abuse involvement and the various phases of the addiction career. There are complex and inter-related influences over time..." NIDA, "Addiction Careers: Summary of Studies Based on the DARP 12-Year Followup," Spring/Summer 1985 (Washington DC: Government Printing Office, 1986).
12. Constance Holden, "Is Alcohol Treatment Effective?" *Science* 236 (April 1987): 20-22.
13. Joseph Mayer and Rebecca Black, "Relationship between Alcoholism and Child Abuse and Neglect," *Currents in Alcoholism, Vol. II,* ed. Frank A. Sexius (New York: Grune and Stratton, 1977).
14. Richard D. Moore, et al., "Prevalence, Detection and Treatment of Alcoholism in Hospitalized Patients," *Journal of the American Medical Association* 261 (1989): 403-7.
15. Paul Haberman and Michael Baden, *Alcohol, Other Drugs and Violent Death* (New York: Oxford, 1978).
16. Board of Trustees Report, "Alcohol: Advertising, Counteradvertising and Depiction in the Media," *Journal of the American Medical Association* 256 (19 September 1986): 1485-88.
17. A pilot study on infants born with drugs in their bloodstream was conducted by the author and Professor Seth Fisher of the Department of Sociology at the University of California at Santa Barbara.
18. Michael D. Newcomb and Peter Bentley, *Consequences of Adolescent Drug Use: Impact on the Lives of Young Adults* (Newbury Park, CA: Sage, 1988).
19. "Debate Resurrected Over Risks of Casual Drug Use," *Los Angeles Times,* 10 August 1988, I 1:1. Newcomb and Bentley's study was a prime source for the *Time"s* article.
20. Ibid., I 20.
21. Ibid.
22. Ibid.
23. James B. Jacobs, "Drinking and Crime," *Crime File Series* (Washington, DC: National Institute of Justice, 1984).
24. John D. Hundley, "Drug Usage and Outstanding Performance Among Young Adolescents," *Addictive Behaviors* 10 (1985): 419-23.
25. "Crime Study Finds Recent Drug Use in Most Arrested," *New York Times,* 22 January 1988, I 1:6. For a review of recent research on drugs and crime, see Bernard Gropper, "Probing the Links Between Drugs and Crime," *National Institute of Justice: Research in Brief* (Washington, DC: National Institute of Justice, 1985).
26. "Doubts Cast on Crime Rates Ties to Drug War," *Los Angeles Times,* 6 September 1991, A 20:1.
27. Fred Holsten, "The Female Drug Abuser: Has She a Shorter Way Out?" *The Journal of Drug Issues* 15 (1985): 391.
28. Ibid.
29. "Surgeon-General Asserts Smoking is an Addiction," *New York Times,* 17 May 1988, I 1:5.

30. Drugs are used either to reduce craving or withdrawal symptoms (an example is the use of methadone for heroin addicts); to treat what is thought to be an underlying depression or psychological problem of some sort (for example, desipramine for cocaine); to block the effects of the drug the person is addicted to or to simply make the person sick if they ingest such a drug (for example, anabuse for individuals addicted to alcohol). From Deborah Barnes, "Breaking the Cycle of Addiction," *Science* 241 (August 1988): 1029-30.

31. Motoi Hayashida, et al. "Comparative Effectiveness and Costs of Inpatient and Outpatient Detoxification of Patients with Mild-to-Moderate Alcohol Withdrawal Syndrome," *New England Journal of Medicine* 320 (9 February 1989): 358-65.

32. Reginald G. Smart, "Do Some Alcoholics Do Better In Some Types of Treatment Than Others?" *Drug and Alcohol Dependence* 3 (1978): 65-75.

33. Ibid.

34. Unpublished research by Dr. Steven Barkley, Medical Director of Cottage Care Hospital, Santa Barbara, CA. This was part of a pilot study on infants born with drugs in their bloodstream performed with a grant provided by the University of California at Santa Barbara to Professor Seth Fisher.

35. "Keys to fighting drugs seen as educating youth, halting supply," *Gallup Report No. 270* (March 1988): 33.

36. "Bennett Scoffs at 'Touchy-Feely' Approach to Drug Prevention," *Los Angeles Times*, 7 March 1990, A 15L1.

37. Mary Ann Pentz, et al., "A Multicommunity Trial for Primary Prevention of Adolescent Drug Abuse," *Journal of the American Medical Association* 261 (9 June 1989): 3259-66.

38. Ibid., 3259.

39. Ibid.

40. Ibid.

41. Eric Schaps, et al., "Evaluation of Seven School-based Prevention Programs: A final report on the Napa Project," *International Journal of the Addictions* 21 (1986): 1081-1112. David Forbes, "Saying No to Ron and Nancy: School-based Drug Abuse Prevention Programs in the 1980's," *Journal of Education* 169 (1987): 81-90 offers a thoughtful opinion on drug education.

42. Richard Blum, *Drug Education: Results and Recommendations* (Lexington, MA: Lexington Books, 1976), 170.

43. Ibid.

44. "Surgeon General Says Children Are Targets of Tobacco Industry," *Los Angeles Times*, 1 June 1990, A 17:1.

45. T. Patrick Macdonald and Rhoda Estep, "Prime Time Drug Depictions," *Contemporary Drug Problems* 12 (Fall 1985): 419-30.

46. Ibid.

6

Current Policy and Contradictions

On 5 September, 1989, George Bush made a major policy speech regarding the Federal effort to relieve the drug crisis. The heart of the speech was a reported increase of $2.2 billion in anti-drug programs. The Federal government was already spending about $6 billion in law enforcement efforts and $600 million in education and drug treatment programs. The announced new expenditures were skewed toward more law enforcement; approximately $1.8 billion more would be spent on it, with drug education and treatment centers receiving some $400 million additional dollars.

These were the facts according to Mr. Bush's much publicized speech. Holding up a bag of crack throughout the speech, Mr. Bush exhorted state and local officials to increase their efforts, including putting more individuals behind bars for a longer period of time. Winding up his speech he stated "...if we face this evil as a nation united, this [referring to the bag of crack] will be nothing but a handful of useless chemicals."[1]

That bag of crack is a relevant story in and of itself. According to news reports, reporters were interested in the origins of the bag and asked how the administration had obtained the "crack." The obvious source would have been the Drug Enforcement Agency, but White House staffers had not used that source. Instead they had gone out on the street and purchased the bag from a local dealer. To further the media potential, they had persuaded the dealer to come to Lafayette Park to make the deal. Hence, the President could claim that such drugs were being sold in the shadow of the White House. After the press had reported the various details, the staffer led local police to the dealer, who was arrested (the staffer was not).[2]

In spite of the sensationalism, and the muddleheadedness of the purchase, and in spite of putting an unaware Mr. Bush in the rather embarrassing position of illegal possession, the ease of purchase of the drug remains a genuine story. The story is relevant because of the special attention the nation's capital has received during the drug crisis. As previously noted, in Washington D.C. there has been a joint effort of Federal and local officials to end the drug crisis through law enforcement. Here all the policies advocated by the White House are in effect: more arrests (a twelvefold increase between 1981 and 1986) more prosecutions (a sevenfold increase), more convictions (a twelvefold increase) and more jail terms (a fourfold increase)(all for the same time period of 1981-1986, the last year of available data).[3] Yet, according to the D.C. police chief, the problem is worse now (drug-related homicides have increased) than before the special effort was implemented.[4] Furthermore, general usage has not declined any more than the national average.[5] This, obviously, was not a theme of Mr. Bush's speech. Instead, he asked for more money for more of the same policy. The policy that failed in D.C. was the policy Mr. Bush advocated for the entire country.

Moreover, the additional funding announced by Mr. Bush was somewhat bogus. Much of the "new" funding was paid for by taking funds away from other social service programs, such as public housing subsidies and juvenile criminal justice programs. Given the embeddedness of the drug crisis in larger social ills, such cutbacks are self-defeating. As one expert noted in the Los Angeles Times: "You give me a 13-year-old who's functionally illiterate, who dropped out of school, has no family, has been hustling on the street...and there's no social, emotional and personal strength to build on, the long-run outcome is quite a bit more dismal."[6]

Yet programs designed to help such youths are precisely the programs Mr. Bush proposed cutting back to pay for more police and more prisons. A further point, beyond the question of how funding is spent, is that a major speech emphasizing "new" funding was deceptive and deliberately so.

The fact is that of the $2.2 billion in "additional" funding, only $716 million represented new funding addressing the drug crisis. The difference between the $2.2 billion announced and the $716 million real increase was from increases that Congress had already voted on that year and the previous year. The drug crisis, already a windfall for the underground market, is at the same time a windfall for political leaders seeking sensational causes, causes in which emotions come before facts, and in which political concerns come before the genuine needs of the public.

Because the actual increase was so much smaller than the real increase, as well as the fact that law enforcement (the politically safe alternative, already heavily funded), was to receive the bulk of the increase, Congress immediately proposed additional increases, with the increases slanted toward education and treatment. The Senate approved a $9.4 billion anti-drug program some two weeks after Mr. Bush's speech, an increase of $1.2 billion over the White House request, with some $800 million of the increase for education and treatment. Mr. Bush, rather than welcoming the Congressional response, angrily denounced the Senate's action and accused the Senate of playing "price-tag politics."[7] Unlike, of course, Mr. Bush's administration.

Even within the administration and within the ranks of law enforcement, political concerns interfere with pursuing the drug crisis. A former cocaine trafficker and money launderer turned government witness pinpointed the problem of the lack of cooperation between the Federal Bureau of Investigation and the DEA. At one point, he was questioned by the DEA about certain drug activities of his and the agents were entirely unaware that he had already provided the information to the FBI some ten months previously. "The FBI won't tell the DEA, the DEA won't tell the FBI and nobody wants to talk to Customs," the informant was quoted as saying. "Everyone has their own budget priorities."[8]

Government officials (in this case, Assistant FBI Director Milton Ahlerich) have defended the restriction upon the exchange of communication as necessary to protect the identity of witnesses.[9] However, such a position is equally damning. What it truly reveals is the degree of mistrust that characterizes interagency relationships. Such mistrust is also actively sustained and encouraged by agency chiefs.

A former prosecutor testifying before Congress disclosed another case about a government at odds with itself. Apparently, U.S. authorities had attempted to apprehend a Colombian drug chief while he was in Venezuela in October 1988. However, the effort was blocked and not by a corrupt foreign government or police department; the effort was blocked by the U.S. Government itself, namely the State Department. A representative from the State Department defended the Department's action by claiming the situation was "more complicated" than what Congress had been told, without, according to the press report, specifying just what that "complication" was.[10]

Moreover, as will be further noted, the Reagan Administration itself deliberately overlooked the drug connections of Central American allies such as Noriega and also Honduran military leaders (as well as others, to be noted later) in exchange for their cooperation in the Contra effort. The Reagan administration, for example, shut down the DEA office in Honduras when the drug connections of the Hondurans became public knowledge. In this way, the Honduran pipeline was deliberately protected.

Aircraft carriers have been stationed off the South American coast; blimps and troops are proposed for the Mexico-United States border; international anti-drug cartels are announced; but all along the U.S. government has protected various cocaine routes into the United States in the name of national security. In the case of the Reagan administration, the deals generally were to protect various cartel members or associated members in exchange for help in supplying the Contras (this occurred after Congress had outlawed military assistance). The amount of cocaine that has been smuggled into the United States with the complicity of the American government is unknown.

There is another critical set of reasons for the failure of law enforcement to mitigate the crisis, despite the billions poured each year into this policy (some $30 billion in Federal expenditures in the years 1986-91):[11] the very nature of the problem on the one hand and then contradictions within the policy itself on the other. These contradictions are argued here to exist in tandem with the political posturing that puts media events before the genuine facts of the "drug crisis."

The very nature of the drug problem limits the effectiveness of law enforcement. The drug problem in all its aspects, tends to be pushed around by law enforcement rather than solved. One police officer put the problem of drugs and enforcement in the following perspective: "It's like pushing an air bubble around inside an air mattress—it changes location but it doesn't go away...[Still] that doesn't mean you don't try to get rid of it."[12]

The officer was referring to the usefulness of temporarily roping off areas of the city, particularly sections hard-hit by drug dealers, but his words are relevant to all aspects of the drug crisis. As noted a number of times, expert advice is available but hardly attended to by legislators and policymakers. As will be seen, the law enforcement option is not rejected in the proposals to be made here, but is rather presented as a last resort.

Close down one street and the action only shifts to another street; close down one town or area, such as Miami and Florida (or at least increase the heat to the extent that smugglers are truly uncomfortable) and the action only shifts to Los Angeles. Then in Los Angeles, the county will become overwhelmed as by the number of drug cases in the courtroom as well as by the number of drug cases pending or awaiting a decision by prosecutors. Turn the heat up in Colombia or Mexico, and the action shifts to the Bahamas, Haiti, Guatemala or even Brazil. Pressure marijuana growers in California and Mexico, and Kentucky becomes a major marijuana growing region. Put out the alarm regarding "crack" and the drug of choice becomes "ice" or "crank," a form of methamphetamine.

For every action taken—understand this means effective action—the sole consequence appears to be that the problem is only displaced somewhere else. This is a clear indication of the limits of effective police action, and a clear indication that police action must be given second priority to measures that get at the underlying conditions generating the drug crisis.

The present policy of making busts and making arrests has had its successes. To recap briefly stories already discussed, there was the seizure of 21 tons of cocaine in a Los Angeles warehouse and the seizure of 9 tons of cocaine in Texas. Also, there has been the arrest and extradition of a number of leaders of the Medellin cartel (by far the most violent of the cocaine cartels). For example, Rafael Munoz Talavera, the owner of the 21 tons of cocaine confiscated in the Sylmar warehouse, was arrested in November 1989. The reputed finance officer of the Medellin cartel was arrested and extradited to the United States in October 1989. A Honduran said to be one of the chief money launderers of the Medellin cartel was convicted in September 1989 in Los Angeles. A second major money launderer, Eduardo Martinez Romero was arrested in the same month. Most notably, Pablo Escobar, the leader of the Medellin cartel, surrendered to Colombian authorities in June 1991.

All these individuals were captured with great difficulty. An added problem is that, like the Prohibition-era gangsters of our history, they were popular among their own people. The Honduran money launderer, Juan Ramon Matta Ballesteros, employed as many as 5,000 people in his various legal businesses and was widely respected and liked in his home region. A more dramatic story is that of Rodriques Gacha (called "El

Mexicano"), the reputed head of the Med cartel who was killed after a 72-hour shoot-out with the American and Columbian military. Similarly, Escobar proved quite popular in his country; U.S. officials were taken aback by the uncritical press treatment given him.

However, despite these successes, estimates are that the flow of marijuana and cocaine has increased into the country, even after an expenditure of $30 billion in Federal law enforcement dollars since 1986. Peter Reuter of RAND Corporation (a Santa Monica based thinktank) undertook the most referenced evaluation of the success of interdiction. To iterate, Reuter found that although seizures had increased from 1.7 tons of cocaine in 1981 to 25 tons of cocaine in 1985, the increases in the supply of cocaine were more than enough to make up the difference. Despite the increased seizures, the price of cocaine has declined from $60,000 a kilo in 1981 to $35,000 in 1986.[13] In fact, the price declined to $15,000 a kilo in 1989 before edging back up.

By 1989, seizures had increased to 160 tons, yet the price was still lower than in 1986. Therefore, law enforcement personnel increased their estimate of world production of cocaine to 700 tons annually, with 550 tons, or 80 percent, of that production going to the U.S. market. However, findings of increasingly diluted cocaine at the street level have given officials some hope of having turned the corner with interdiction. Yet, a reading of Reuter's report leads one to suspect that this optimism is considerably premature.

Reuter maintains that interdiction success is bound to be elusive, given the number of suppliers and supply routes into the United States. Therefore, to Reuter, the real question is how the interdiction program affects the risks and costs to underground marketeers. This was the question Reuter was asked to address by the Defense Department (back when the Defense Department was less enthusiastic about taking part in the war on drugs). Reuter estimates that only 5 percent of the retail price of cocaine accounts for all smuggling costs. This means that smugglers can lose a cocaine shipment to law enforcement agencies and readily replace that shipment, given the low cost of what was lost relative to the profit on the next shipment.[14]

Furthermore, he calculates that a tripling of the leaf price (estimating the effect of interdiction at the location where coca leaf is grown) would add no more than 1 percent to the retail cost of cocaine (again, given the low costs of the raw material). He estimates that if seizures were to increase from 20 percent (the government's estimate of its interdiction success) to 50 percent of all cocaine imported into the country, the effect would be to add less than 3 percent to the retail price of cocaine.[15] Reuter's estimates of the risk of arrest are similarly in favor of the smugglers. In fact, he estimates that the risks fell between the years 1981 and 1985.[16] This is true despite a two and a half times increase in law enforcement expenditures between the years 1981 and 1985 (no later estimates of risks are available).

However, the reasons for the failure of domestic law enforcement cannot be understood solely on the basis of the nature of the problem. At a higher level of policy, we find extraordinary contradictions that if continued are guaranteed to doom the law enforcement effort—no matter how many billions are thrown at the problem. These contradictions are fourfold: first, briefly repeated here, there is the contradiction of what is *not* proposed by the current administration. There are any number of options that would point toward the mitigation of the "drug crisis," options that would not cost the taxpayer a single dollar, yet these options are never voiced by current authorities because of the political costs involved in proposing them.

For example, the most widely abused drug is alcohol. Advertising for this drug is pervasive; it is estimated that the industry spends some $1.2 billion a year promoting this particular drug. Moreover, such ads are the staple of sports programming, a programming particularly popular with young people. Further, the industry spends some $20 million a year promoting drinking by young people via advertising in college newspapers, concerts, etc. It would seem prudent, if one was sincerely interested in reducing the nation's drug crisis, to ban such ads. Yet not a word about restricting such ads is heard from public officials.

The story is the same with tobacco. Alcohol and tobacco are powerful industries, generous to both political parties and richly rewarded for their generosity by being ignored in the "war against drugs." Of course, these are the drugs of the mainstream medicine society, whatever their genuine danger, and mainstream drugs historically have received protection from the recurrent "wars." When they have not, such as during Prohibition, the response was no different than today's response: many who preferred the drug simply ignored the law. The response of public officials was to push the law enforcement option harder, the result then being the same as now: the creation of an underground market with all the resulting problems of official and police corruption, as well as the empowerment of the most violent and lawless aspects of American society.

The second contradiction is the familiar and typical problem of bureaucratic infighting: the FBI does not talk to the DEA and vice versa. Each regards the drug war as their turf and each is suspicious of the other agency's ability to keep information confidential. The peculiar response of the Bush administration has been to propose that the agencies be further split. At present, the DEA reports to the FBI director (in theory this is so, but it has not been the practice); a current proposal suggests that the DEA become an entirely independent agency. It is difficult to see how this will improve communications and cooperation, which are the reasons given for the proposal.

Then we have an administration that loudly scolds the rest of the world (and anyone and anything that might make any sort of a respectable target, including state legislators) for their lack of effort in the drug war, while the same government overlooks the role of giant corporations such as Exxon and Shell in the underground market. These two corporations supply the underground market with the chemicals necessary to convert the coca leaf to cocaine.[17] Meanwhile, the government arrests the owners of mom-and-pop type horticultural stores for supplying equipment that might be used to grow marijuana.

The Federal government has the power to stop the shipment of chemicals used in the drug trade. After the participation of Exxon and Shell became public knowledge, the Bush administration acted by banning shipments to some South American companies but only to a small percentage of those receiving the chemicals. Therefore, the profits of the oil companies were protected and a front page story could be produced on how the administration had finally acted. Buried in the back pages was the story of just how shaky was the so-called ban.[18]

Likewise, the Reagan and the Bush administrations have refused to endorse legislation that would make money laundering more difficult. The argument of the Bush administration is that such legislation would interfere with the money operations of legitimate businesses. The problem is that such money operations are, when not illegal, done simply to deprive the U.S. Treasury of tax income, not something one would think an administration would protect.[19]

In short, there is the contradiction of protecting the practices that the underground market needs in order to maintain a smooth production and financing flow. This is the third contradiction of policy. This could be alternatively understood as busting the politically unconnected while ignoring the more harmful practices of well-heeled and influential American corporations.

There is a fourth contradiction, the critical contradiction: the active protection of the drug pipeline into the United States and the cooperation with various players in the drug market in exchange for their continuing support of the American anti-communist effort. This protection to cartel members and associates is provided even as the military with, once again, great trumpeting, is sent into the so-called "war against drugs," an effort that included the proposal to send carriers into the Caribbean to hunt down drug smugglers. Such protection is offered to drug smugglers even as speech after speech is delivered by administration members against the evils of drugs and the drug cartels.

The details of this story, the story of the largest and most dangerous member of the drug cartels—the U.S. government during the administrations of Reagan/Bush will now be provided. The primary reference is the Kerry (Senator John Kerry, D-Mass.) subcommittee report on the Reagan/Bush administration's cooperation with drug cartel members and organizations.[20] A major source for the Kerry subcommittee was the testimony of Richard Gregorie. Mr. Gregorie is a former federal prosecutor and head of the anti-drug effort in Miami who resigned in protest over the government's obstruction of its own drug investigations and prosecutions.

Oliver North, the State Department, and the DEA in Central America

A good way to undermine the effectiveness of anti-cartel efforts would be to enter into contracts with cartel members to supply illegal goods to American allies (such as military supplies to the Contras, a supply operation that had been outlawed by Congress). Another good way to keep the drug pipeline open is to look the other way when the drug smugglers that one has contracted with continue smuggling drugs as well. Indeed, one might even prevent their arrest by other government agencies on the basis of the aid they have provided. When all else fails, one might even close down any law enforcement offices one has in their country, thereby preventing any chance of anyone getting arrested. This is the story of the U.S. government in Central America during the Reagan/Bush years.

The stories of Oliver North's operations and the perplexing protection of Panama's Noriega by, of all agencies, the DEA, have
received some attention in the press. At the same time the connections between Noriega and Bush have also received some attention, with the question raised as to why Mr. Bush continued to
meet with and defend Noriega after Noriega's association with the
drug cartels became public knowledge (or at least government
knowledge).[21]

However, what is overlooked is that such cooperation with cartel
members and allies was not the exception but rather the general
rule of American policy. The significance of this larger context is
that such protection of various key players and drug pipelines into
the United States could well be continuing today. This would be
extraordinarily hypocritical, yet no less hypocritical than what has
already occurred. For example, in 1986, the State Department contracted with four different Central American companies to deliver
supplies to the Contras. All four companies were run by cartel
members or associates. Yet, even after being informed by the FBI
that the companies were run by underground marketeers, the State
Department continued the contracts.[22] Likewise, Oliver North's
Contra supply effort involved working with known drug
smugglers.[23] Why?

A quote from General Paul Gorman, head of American military
forces in the region, becomes relevant: "If you want to move arms
or munitions in Latin America, the established networks are
owned by the cartels. It has lent itself to the purposes of terrorists,
of saboteurs, of spies, of insurgents, and of subversives."[24]

Apparently, this is why Reagan/Bush personnel worked with
cartel personnel in the Contra supply effort. The drug cartels,
because of their business-like and also ruthless management of
that market, were evidently the most dependable and effective
organizations in Central America and the Caribbean. White House
personnel, such as Oliver North (but not only North), may have
had nowhere else to turn if they were to successfully get arms to
the Contras.

Of course, this was contrary to the law and North's heroic image
after deceiving a Congressional investigation is hardly understandable. Nonetheless, it is also clear he was given a specific
assignment from higher up (North claims from CIA Director
William Casey, but the evidence is not clear), and equally clear
that foreign policy matters often occur in shadow, under secret
orders, and often are thought beyond the law. Moreover, the DEA

itself cooperated with drug marketeers, the most notable being Noriega of Panama. As early as 1983 a National Security Council member described the accumulated evidence of Noriega's drug market involvement as "...not a 'smoking gun' but rather a twenty-one gun cannon barrage of evidence."[25]

However, five years later, DEA Chief John Lawn was testifying before Congress of Noriega's long history of cooperation with the DEA. Furthermore, in 1986, the DEA chief wrote a letter to Noriega expressing Lawn's "...deep appreciation for the vigorous anti-drug trafficking policy that you have adopted, which is reflected in the numerous expulsions from Panama of accused traffickers."[26] But the evidence indicates that Noriega was using his liaison with the DEA as a cover under which to continue his drug market activities. Noriega, a throwback to the days of banana dictatorships, was also (and at the same time of Lawn's letter) the cartel's man in Panama. Hence Noriega was successfully able to work both sides of the street: letters of commendation from the DEA and profits from permitting the drug cartels to use Panama as a drug transit and money laundering center. Furthermore, Noriega's work was not independent of Panama's government. Rather, the police and military, as well as the financial institutions of Panama, were all put in the service of Noriega and the cartels.[27]

Noriega was only the most famous of the drug marketeers to work both sides of the street. North's Contra supply operation also proved useful to drug marketeers seeking protection from drug busts. Drug marketeers were astute enough to recognize that participating in Contra resupply efforts would provide them with a White House willing to speak up for them were they ever arrested for their drug activities. So, under the cover of resupplying the Contras, their drug smuggling could continue, this time with an insurance policy against arrest.[28]

Indeed, they were right. The DEA itself blocked prosecutions for drug-runners turned informants, even when other agencies felt it was the drug-runner using the DEA and not vice-versa.[29] Arranging to "work" with one arm of the government in order to prevent prosecution by another arm was called "ticket-punching." It was insurance against arrest and apparently it worked rather well for a number of drug marketeers.[30]

North's operations are over but the DEA's continues, as yet unscrutinized by the press and unnoticed by the public. Such illogical practices ensure a government tripping over its own feet and perhaps explains why the FBI prefers to distance itself from the operations of the DEA.

In Central America, every player—the DEA, North, the cartels, Noriega—was working both sides of the street. In the Machiavellian tangle of snares and countersnares that followed, weaker players such as Noriega and lower level officials such as North were shut down. The stronger players, U.S. drug enforcement agencies and the cartels, remain. The effect of escalating the war (and all sides playing both sides of the street) was that the weaker participants were winnowed out. Perhaps this is an indication of what will happen within the United States as the "war against drugs" continues to escalate. The net effect will be to do the dirty work of the stronger "gangs," clearing the field of weaker competitors and thereby increasing the market and the profits of the strongest and most violent.

The Caribbean

Panama and Colombia dominate the headlines but the refinement, transportation, and money laundering activities of the underground market hardly stop there. Other Central and South American countries participate; for example the military governments of Honduras and Paraguay and possibly Guatemala. In Honduras, as has been noted, after the involvement of the Honduran military in the drug trade became public knowledge, the DEA heroically responded by shutting down its one office in the country.

Evidently, the Honduran officials are protected because of their helpfulness in assisting the Contra resupply effort. "It wasn't that there was a cover-up," said one administration figure quoted in the New York Times. "It's that people knew certain questions shouldn't be asked."[31] This, of course, is "ticket-punching" on a larger scale.

In addition, the island nations of the Caribbean, smuggling nations since the time of European colonization, and tax/financial havens since the advent of modern finance, perform such traditional services for the drug marketeers as well. In the case of underground financial services, this is something mainstream American businesses and clients turn to also. This is another example of how the underground market is intertwined with the visible, legal market and how the "drug crisis" has its roots in accepted mainstream practices.

In the Bahamas, money is accepted with no questions asked. Once the money is deposited into an offshore account, individuals and organizations of the above or underground market, can then readily transfer the money into the United States. Once in the United States, the money is available for investment in stocks, bonds, real estate, whatever. This is a critical service that the drug marketeers could not accomplish without help from the mainstream.

Greenbacks are liquid only in small amounts. Drug marketeers need a mechanism for getting their cash into a bank account without tripping regulations that require banks to report transactions of over $10,000. This is not to say that banks always follow such laws; the Bank of Boston and Bank of America are two banks who were sanctioned for failure to report such transactions.[32] With U.S. banks under close scrutiny, the business does not end. Instead, typically for the drug market, the business simply changes location. Banks in the Bahamas (and previously, Noriega's banks) simply received more of the business than before.

The law enforcement effort in the Bahamas is the same as previously noted in Central America: the government and the drug marketeers seek to play both sides of the street. Only in the Bahamas, it is the DEA that seeks to straightforwardly pressure the government of the Bahamas and it is the State Department (possibly with the American military's blessing) that is protecting the underground market. There is a U.S. military base in the Bahamas and the drug activities of members of the government of the Bahamas took a back seat to the negotiations over the base.

The State Department, over the objections of the DEA, certified the Bahamas as being in "full cooperation" with the war on drugs. The treaty renewing base rights was successfully signed. The basis of the State Department's opinion was a tough anti-drug market law enacted in 1986. However, two years later, only one person, a police officer, had ever been arrested under the law.[33] Nor does the market stop with the Bahamas. There is evidence that Haiti is fast being drawn into the cartel's network. The poverty and disorganization of Haiti, perhaps a country in name only, makes this island a fit refuge for the cartels if the effort to drive them out of the Bahamas becomes more successful.[34]

Castro and Drugs

The American government is not alone in its compromises, denials, and general folly; the actions of the communist government of Cuba parallel those of the United States. Castro is very much anti-drug at home, but he is willing to work with drug marketeers, evidently as part as his anti-American posture. Even as Mr. Bush is willing to work with Noriega in order to further the anti-communist campaigns of the United States, so too is Castro willing to work with the cartels to further his anti-American interests.[35]

Castro's involvement appears to be twofold. First of all, Cuban waters are evidently open to cartel smuggling. Second, Castro has reportedly intervened at least twice to mediate disputes between left-wing guerrillas and the cartels, and then to mediate a dispute between Noriega and the cartels. Castro vehemently denies all such involvement.[36]

Beyond the specifics already detailed, the overall story appears to be one of an organization (the American government) losing sight of its goals. Moreover, the government, given the many aspects of the underground market and the many departments with a hand in drug policy and enforcement, is easily led into arrangements that defeat both. In addition, and consistent with the general hysteria, there appears to be a certain "war mentality" evident in government action, the result being that the interdiction of drugs becomes secondary to "getting them." This is self-defeating and yet it remains today's policy.

For example, there was the manhunt for "El Mexicano," Rodriques Gacha, reputed head of the Medellin cartel.[37] Colombian officials described "El Mexicano" as a "bad apple," a ruthless killer of the innocent and public enemy number one. However, the people who know the man, the "innocent" who should have been seeking government help to protect themselves from the man, instead defended him. Indeed, it was because this man was well-liked that he was so hard to pin down. Government forces nearly caught up with him a number of times, but he was always tipped off by residents and helped to escape. He was reportedly a national celebrity whose friends included the national police and military officers. In his hometown, an intelligence officer was quoted as saying, "He had the sympathy of a majority of the town."[38]

The details of his death are worth noting. From early reports, besides Gacha, there was his 17-year-old son and some five bodyguards. All were killed by some 1,000 police and troops backed by helicopters.[39] At that, it took this small army some 72 hours to dispatch Gacha's small group. Their bodies were buried in paupers' graves without being marked and, possibly, without final sacraments. Mr. Bush, a week before Christmas, pronounced himself "delighted" with the death.[40] This is folk hero material, much as many Prohibition "public enemies" were also folk heroes who became legends following their deaths.

Last and most important to the point made here, American officials admitted that while efforts were focused upon Gacha, the flow of cocaine resumed its previous high levels after some success in disrupting the traffic. Officials deliberately put greater emphasis upon capturing Gacha than on cocaine interdiction. They considered such priorities a necessary price to pay. But such priorities also offer a clue that the drug war is developing its own logic, with drug interdiction taking second place to the war as a war.

In addition, given the tangle of goals and means in the various competing American policies in Central America, anti-communist goals have been equally compromised. For example, in defending and protecting Noriega, American agencies were also protecting Noriega's arms trade activities, including selling arms to left-wing organizations in Central America.[41]

Generally, the cartels are anti-communist. Indeed, the Medellin cartel came about in response to pressure from Colombia's left-wing, the M-19 movement. Previously, various organizations had gone from marijuana smuggling to cocaine smuggling, taking over the cocaine trade in the 1970s in a bloody war called the "Cocaine War."[42] After this, their greatest enemy was the left-wing revolutionaries of the country, who actively sought to put the drug organizations out of business. The various organizations met in Medillin, Colombia (hence their name), and agreed to unify to destroy the movement. They were successful.[43]

However, in the warp and weave of Central American politics, cartel associates such as Noriega, in the arms trade side of their underground business, are suppliers to the left. In addition, in Colombia (after the defeat of M-19) and Peru, left-wing movements are now allies of the underground market. Every group, whatever their size and whatever their legitimacy, involved in the underground market and chaotic politics of the region is also enmeshed in remarkable contradictions and hypocrisies.

Regarding contradictions, the American media itself is not blameless. The media too often acts not as a public watchdog nor even as a detached observer but rather as an enthusiastic cheer-leader of government policy. Hence, rather than exposing contra-dictions to public debate, the media lends itself to government purposes by ignoring and hence burying the debatable facts.

An article, "Narco-Terrorism: A Tale of Two Stories," on the gulli-bility of media coverage appeared in the *Columbian Journalism Review* by Joel Millman.[44] In March 1986, Ronald Reagan made a speech accusing the Sandinista government of drug-running. The evidence presented was rather bare, but the American media hap-pily jumped on the bandwagon and widely reported Mr. Reagan's accusation as proven fact. However, what they did not report was that the DEA itself did not believe the Sandinistas were working with the drug cartels. Indeed, when asked, the DEA noted it had repeatedly stated that there was no connection between the Sandinistas and the cartels and, after Mr. Reagan's remarks, made its position known again "to refute" Mr. Reagan. Ironically, an agency of the Reagan administration was far more critical of Mr. Reagan's remarks than the American press, the self-proclaimed watchdogs of the public interest.[45]

Of course, as previously noted, the American government itself has worked with the drug cartels, most closely during the Contra resupply effort. Further, the Contras themselves were revealed to have been engaged in drug-running into the United States. However, this story was only released by the Associated Press after much foot-dragging and some watering down of the original story by reporters Robert Parry and Brian Barger. Few American papers and none of the television networks picked up on the AP story.

Indeed, the New York Times, when it finally covered the story, headlined not the evidence of drug-running but the denial of such by a "senior official." The Times gave the Contras a clean bill of health based solely upon the word of that official. It was not until six months after the story initially broke that the statehouse press followed up with stories corroborating the initial evidence of Contra drug-running and U.S. complicity. Such a press is certainly a factor in the ineffectiveness of American drug policy, given that such a press so readily covers up and protects official foul-ups and contradictions.

Thus, there are two critical reasons for the failure of law enforcement to deal with the drug crisis: the nature of the prob-lem, a problem that is perpetually displaced but never solved by the application of police force, and then contradictions within the policy itself. Such contradictions are found in the permitting of promotions that encourage the consumption of legal drugs; bureaucracies working at cross-purposes; and ignoring the role of big business in supplying the drug trade with needed chemicals while arresting the politically unconnected. All are stumbling blocks preventing a successful policy.

The largest contradiction of all creates doubts the Federal government genuinely supports its own "war against drugs," the evidence of government compliance in bringing illegal drugs into the country. That such compliance exists is evidence that the government itself suspects its own drug war propaganda. Such skepticism is rarely seen in the press who, for the most part, have been partners in pushing a painless if hysterical view of the war.

Nonetheless, it is also true that newspapers such as the New York Times and Los Angeles Times and certainly others have also covered the other side and views of the "war." Still, while particular articles can be found that bring out the criticisms of the "war," such articles are the exception. Generally, the press is happy to take government and police pronouncements at face value rather than challenge the status quo.

Notes

1. "Bush Tells Plan to Combat Drugs," *Los Angeles Times*, 6 September 1989, A 1:5.
2. "Keystone Kops Drug Buy Near White House Mocked," *Los Angeles Times,* 16 December 1989, A 30:1. A more extensive report of the purchase comes from: Jefferson Morley, "The Kid Who Sold Crack to the President," *Washington City Paper*, 15-21 December 1989.
3. Peter Reuter, et al., *Drug Use and Drug Programs in the Washington Metropolitan Area*, R-3655-GWRC (Santa Monica: RAND Corporation, July 1988), 52.
4. "Reality Intrudes on Drug Crusade in Capital," *New York Times*, 20 October 1989, I 1:3. See also, "U.S. Anti-Drug Effort Called Wrong for D.C.," *The Washington Post*, 16 December 1989.
5. "Reality Intrudes on Drug Crusade in Capital," *New York Times*, 20 October 1989, I 1:3.
6. Quote attributed to Jeff Kushner, director of Oregon's Office of Alcohol and Drug Abuse Programs in "Plan Assailed as Not Aiding All Who Want Treatment," *Los Angeles Times*, 6 September 1989, 11.
7. "White House Calls Byrd Plan Price-Tag Politics," *Los Angeles Times*, 28 September 1989, I 25:1.
8. "Interagency Rivalries Said to Hinder Drug Fight," *Los Angeles Times*, 18 August 1989, I 18:1.

9. Ibid., I 18.

10. Ibid.

11. Additionally, in 1989 alone, states and federal governments spent some $5 billion on prison construction. "Big Catch: Drug War's Little Fish," *Los Angeles Times*, 6 May 1990, A 1:1.

12. Quote attributed to Lt. Gary Rogness, head of LAPD narcotics field enforcement unit in the San Fernando Valley, in "Effectiveness of Roping Off Drug Areas Questioned," *Los Angeles Times*, 18 November 1987, II 1:1.

13. Peter Reuter, Gordon Crawford and Jonathan Cave, *Sealing the Borders*, R-3594-USDP (Washington, DC: RAND National Defense Research Institute, 1988).

14. From a prepared statement by Peter Reuter of RAND Corporation to the House of Representatives Committee on Government Operations, 17 October 1989.

15. Ibid., 79.

16. Ibid.

17. "Cocaine Has a Made in the U.S.A. Label," *Los Angeles Times*, 5 December 1989.

18. "U.S. Acts to Curb Exports of Drug-Making Solvents," *Los Angeles Times*, 6 February 1990, I 21:1. The quantities involved are huge, for example, in August and September 1989, 2.06 million gallons of one chemical alone was shipped into Colombia (methyl ethyl ketone or MEK, a solvent, one of some six key chemicals needed to convert the leaf to cocaine crystals. The other chemicals are acetone, kerosene, sulfuric acid, potassium permanganate, and salts. This chemical has other purposes, specifically for producing rubber cement. However, Colombia has no such industry. See also, "Cocaine Has a Made in the U.S.A. Label."

A curious situation arises that has the American Navy and Coast Guard patrolling Caribbean waters in search of cocaine smugglers, assisted by Air Force AWAC's reconnaissance planes, backed up by thousands of federal, state and local law officers, all seeking to shut down the cocaine trade, while American firms legally sell to Colombian traffickers all they need to make the stuff. Such remarkable official inconsistency shreds the border as certainly as any individual or gang cleverness in bringing the cocaine in.

Spokespersons from the firms involved in selling the cocaine-making chemicals claim to be shocked that such a thing could be happening and express the to-be-expected concern. However, they also claim, "if it were too difficult to get them [the chemicals] from the United States, our customers might just get them from another source" (Garrity Baker, Chemical Manufacturer's Association director of international affairs, "U.S. Acts to Curb Exports of Drug-Making Solvents," *Los Angeles Times*, 6 February 1990, I 21:1).

Such thinking carried the day until October 1989, when a new law, the Chemical Diversion and Trafficking Act, took effect, requiring the shipment of these chemicals to be reported to the DEA and empowering federal authorities to block such shipments. It remains to be seen how severe official action will be. As of the end of 1989, two shipments of chemicals had been blocked. Neither were to Colombia. One was a shipment of acetone to Mexico, the other was a shipment of chemicals to Taiwan.

Before the passage of the new law, federal policy was characterized by flagrant inconsistency, an inconsistency that undermined the effort to mitigate the drug crisis via law enforcement. The inconsistenies of the law enforcement approach does not stop there. In a splendid, if somewhat harmless, example of conspicuous excess, federal drug agents, in October of 1989, arrested 119 people in 46 states for selling horticultural equipment. The DEA claims that the equipment was being used to grow marijuana indoors.

Domestic growers account for 25 percent of the supply of the marijuana market, Colombia produces 40 percent, Mexico 25 percent, and other countries 10 percent ("119 Seized in drive to halt indoor marijuana growing," *New York Times*, 27 October 1989). One has a curious example here: millions of tons of chemicals produced by Shell and Exxon and used in producing cocaine are ignored by federal officials, but they crack down on horticultural stores. Such remarkable inconsistency undermines the law enforcement approach as surely as putting political concerns first.

19. "A Torrent of Dirty Dollars," *Time*, 18 December 1989, 50-56.
20. U.S. Congress, Senate Subcommittee on Narcotics, Terrorism and International Operations, *Drugs, Law Enforcement and Foreign Policy: A Report of the Subcommittee on Narcotics, Terrorism and International Operations*, 13 April 1989, 71-96. This subcommittee was headed by Senator John Kerry of Massachusetts.
21. "Bush and Noriega: Examination of Their Ties," *New York Times*, 27 September 1988, I 1:2. See also, "Officials Say Bush Heard '85 Charge Against Noriega," *New York Times*, 8 May 1988, I1:3.
22. U.S. Congress, Senate Subcommittee on Narcotics, Terrorism and International Operations, *Drugs, Law Enforcement and Foreign Policy*, 114-30.
23. Ibid., 351-52. See also: Leslie Cockburn, *Out of Control: The Story of the Reagan Administration's Secret War in Nicaragua, the Illegal Arms Pipeline, and the Contra Drug Connection* (New York: The Atlantic Monthly Press, 1987).
24. Kerry Subcommittee, *Drugs, Law Enforcement and Foreign Policy*, 31.
25. Statement by Dr. Norman Bailey in testimony before the House Select Committee on Narcotics Abuse and Control, "U.S. Foreign Policy and International Narcotics Control—Part II, SCNAC-100-2-3, 29 March 1988 in U. S. Congress, Senate Subcommittee on Narcotics, Terrorism and International Operations, *Drugs, Law Enforcement and Foreign Policy*, 240.
26. Kerry Subcommittee, *Drugs, Law Enforcement and Foreign Policy*, 246.
27. Ibid., 219-20.
28. Ibid., 331-54.
29. See "The Case of Michael Palmer," in U.S. Congress, Senate Subcommittee

on Narcotics, Terrorism and International Operations, *Drugs, Law Enforcement and Foreign Policy*, 335-41.

30. Ibid., 332.

31. "Fighting Narcotics: U.S. is Urged to Shift Tactics," *New York Times*, 10 April 1988, I 10.

32. See U.S. Congress, Senate Subcommittee on Narcotics, Terrorism and International Operations, *Drugs, Law Enforcement and Foreign Policy*, 302.

33. Ibid., 39-70.

34. Ibid., 185-95.

35. Ibid., 165-85.

36. The Federal government's role in drug trafficking in Central America in the late 1980s was of a lesser sort than in Southeast Asia. In Vietnam the CIA actively assisted in the transport and financing of the drug trade; in Central America, the political and military operations were headed by Oliver North and his activities in regard to cocaine trafficking consisted of simply looking the other way. Of course, given that North spent several days in the White House destroying documentation of his activities, there remains the possibility of a more active involvement in the drug trade. The most often referenced literature on CIA and heroin in Southeast Asia is Alfred E. McCoy, Cathleen B. Read, and Leonard P. Adams II, *The Politics of Heroin in Southeast Asia* (New York: Harper and Row, 1972).

    A more recent work on the CIA's involvement in the drug trade is provided by *Wall Street Journal* reporter Jonathan Kwitny, *Crimes of Patriots: A True Tale of Dope, Dirty Money and the CIA* (New York: W. W. Norton, 1987). For a further report on the Latin American drug trade see Scott B. Macdonald, *Dancing on a Volcano* (New York: Praeger, 1988). MacDonald's work does not present or discuss evidence of the American government's involvement in the drug trade, however, with that important exception, it provides a first-rate review of reports from Latin-America. The most incisive report on the Reagan Administration's role in the drug trade is by Leslie Cockburn, *Out of Control: The Story of the Reagan Administration's Secret War in Nicaragua, the Illegal Arms Pipeline, and the Contra Drug Connection* (New York: The Atlantic Monthly Press, 1987).

37. "Colombian Police Kill Drug Lord," *Los Angeles Times*, 16 December 1989, A 1:6.

38. Ibid., A 20.

39. "Bloody Killing of Cocaine Kingpin Fills Colombia with Glee, Tension," *Los Angeles Times*, 17 December 1989, A7:1. This is a misleading headline given the content of that and other stories about Gacho.

40. "Bush Says He's Delighted by Death of Notorious Colombian Drug Lord," *Los Angeles Times*, 17 December 1989, A 6:1.

41. U.S. Congress, Senate Subcommittee on Narcotics, Terrorism and International Operations, *Drugs, Law Enforcement and Foreign Policy*, 212-58.

42. Ibid, 71-96.
43. Ibid., 77.
44. Joel Millman, "Narco-terroism: A tale of two stories," *Columbian Journalism Review* 25 (Sept/Oct 1986): 48-51.
45. Ibid., 49.

Part Three
An Alternative Policy

7

Current Policy, Underground

Markets, and Prisons

The last chapter explained the failings of a law enforcement approach in terms of the "drug crisis" and in terms of the contradictions within the law enforcement option. This chapter begins the work of constructing an alternative approach.

The first task must be to understand the consequences of the law enforcement option—quite apart from its failure. These consequences can be understood as the secondary effects of the "drug crisis," effects created by the laws themselves.

The first such effect to be examined is the creation of an underground market in desired goods. A second consequence is the direct effect of enforcement of the drug laws—the filling of court dockets and prisons. The third set of effects is at the level of policy—the increase of government authority at the expense of individual liberty. It must also be understood how these interact at the street level.

If absolute legalization is rejected, then our task is to specify the regulations that would improve current conditions. Any regulations must be enforced and hence the problem of law enforcement remains critical. To rightfully construct an alternative policy, the secondary consequences, the effects created by the drug laws themselves, must be made thoroughly explicit for the warning they will supply.

The law enforcement approach to the drug crisis creates an underground market. The creation of such a market leads to the formation of "gangs" to supply and profit from the existence of that market. The creation of gangs inevitably leads to violence. This violence, at first directed at other gangs, inevitably spills over into attacks upon innocent bystanders.

There is nothing new in this story, though current policymakers appear oblivious to these social facts. Nor will the ending be new, the construction of organized crime groups that will continue to prey upon and penetrate ever deeper the aboveground market and streets. Once such groups form, they remain. The realistic goal then becomes their containment.

So the law enforcement approach not only fails, it makes the problem worse by bringing with it all the problems that the creation of an underground market brings. As has been pointed out, if a pre-*perestroika* Soviet Union could not shut down its own internal underground market it is far-fetched to maintain that the United States can solely using the tools of law enforcement.

Certainly not all prohibited goods produce an underground market of appreciable size, but drugs always have (60 percent of the world's production of illicit drugs is for the American market). A question to be addressed later is—how much demand is produced by the prohibition itself?

Regarding the problems generated by such markets: first, these underground markets, by definition illegitimate, are controlled by individuals who are prepared to use violence to protect and promote their interests and who have little or no interest in the welfare of the community. Furthermore, the existence of the underground market becomes a source of strength to these individuals, financing their predilections and, paradoxically, by filling their pockets with profits, making these individuals figures of respect within the very same neighborhoods whose health and welfare they are undermining.

One might be tempted to have some sympathy for the leaders of these gangs. After all, their lives are considered disposable by the powers that be, the governmental authorities that begrudge providing underclass youth with the basics of food and health care and who provide only the semblance of an education and public services to such neighborhoods. In addition, one might even balance the violence of such gangs against police violence and the lack of constitutional protections that plague such underclass areas.

However, such sympathy would overlook the fact that these gangs have no more concern for the neighborhood than do the powers-that-be. Gangs prey on underclass neighborhoods, contributing to the street violence that was already a massive problem, poisoning young lives and taking away whatever chance there might be for upward mobility and a better life. In addition, and parallel to the legal market, gangs make profits their first and foremost goal regardless of social consequences.

Nonetheless, what is also true is that even as underclass neighborhoods are feeling the extreme side of a law enforcement policy, so too are underclass "gangs" particularly singled out for police and media attention. In fact, there are all sorts of ethnic "gangs," many of whom are not involved in the drug trade. Still, what has set the underclass gangs apart from the rest is the public violence they engage. It is this violence that has drawn both police and media attention.

Put more exactly, the public violence that occurs outside their neighborhood attracts this attention. For example, Los Angeles area gangs did not become notorious until a woman was killed in the upper-middle class neighborhood of Westwood. But such violence is still less than that suffered in the neighborhoods. Moreover, violence is only one sort of cost the marketeers impose.

High school athletes in underclass neighborhoods are highly esteemed individuals to their peers and to youths. A football coach at an underclass high school defined the virtues of such athletes: "They can get things done...they're used to following orders and being on a team. And once they commit to a team they're used to going all out."[1] All the virtues associated with sports participation are virtues that could serve such individuals well in the legitimate business world, but these virtues are instead applied to gang participation.

A recent report indicates that gangs are going out of their way to recruit such athletes. In the northeast section of the San Fernando Valley, police estimated that some 25 former athletes had joined the area's drug and gang scene. Salaries are high, estimated at $1500 a week. Such salaries are offered individuals who, despite their virtues, have few prospects for success when college scholarships are not forthcoming. A further bonus is that such athletes treat their bodies well and are highly disciplined. Hence, despite news stories that sensationalize drug use by athletes, they are less likely than other individuals to use drugs even when such drugs are easily available. This makes them yet more valuable to such gangs.

These individuals are the hope of their families and communities and, in addition, such individuals could do well in the mainstream business community. Instead, they become part of the problem. If American businesses wanted to contribute to solving the drug crisis in the underclass, perhaps a good place to start would be to find employment for such youths: the qualities instilled by participation in athletics could be given equal consideration with grades by American businesses.

Of course, quite apart from athletes, there are plenty of stories of young people from the underclass seizing the opportunity offered by the underground market. For example, there are stories of 12-year-olds earning $300/day in the cocaine/crack business. One such story was featured in the *Los Angeles Times*. The mother of one 12-year-old youth described the positive difference the drug money had meant to her and her son. The mother, a woman with cancer, also fears she will outlive her son.[2]

Nonetheless, these reports beg the question of whether such stories are the exception or the rule. Peter Reuter of RAND (this is the same individual who did the research for the government on the effects of interdiction and the results of government policy in Washington, D.C.) has provided the most detailed and thoroughly researched facts about "dealing."[3]

According to Reuter, some 40 percent of dealers earn approximately $3,000 a month, another 40 percent earn approximately $1,200 dollars a month, and the rest earn about $200 or less a month. Three-quarters of dealers have a job in the mainstream, though their earnings are less than $850 a month. Dealing is described as a supplement to their income, a "second job" sort of activity.[4] In other words, most dealers are otherwise respectable citizens working at full-time jobs, no doubt earning much of their under the table income by selling to other respectable, fully employed friends at work.

Another question becomes the extent of gang involvement in the drug trade. According to a study by two University of Southern California researchers, Malcolm W. Klein and Cheryl L. Maxson: "The world of rock cocaine ["crack," the smokable and cheap form of cocaine] belongs principally to the normal drug dealers of Los Angeles, not to its street gangs."[5]

These researchers found that of all drug traffickers arrested in 1988, only 25 percent of those arrested were gang members. Hence, the gang role should not be minimized but it should be put into perspective. Gangs are a minority in drug trafficking: if all drug marketeering by gangs were stopped, the drug market would go on with minimal disruption. The researchers further estimated that of the 70,000 Black, Latino, and Asian gang members in Los

Angeles, some 10,000 were involved in the underground market in drugs. This is not a trivial number but, at the same time, there is more going on with these gangs than the drug trade. The data base of this study was 741 cocaine arrests in 1984 and 1985 in the Los Angeles area.

Two months after this study, another came out that contradicted the previous interpretation. The second report maintained that gang members are less likely to be arrested because of an elaborate communications network and that gang members may conceal their memberships when they are arrested. This study was done by Jerome H. Skolnick, a researcher at the Center for the Study of Law and Society at UC Berkeley.[6]

This latter report was publicized by the California Attorney General who explicitly compared it to the earlier report and stated (in the *Los Angeles Times*): "Our concern is that the first report minimizes the connection between gangs and drugs.... We believe gangs are very important in the drug trafficking business."[7] The data base was considerably smaller than the earlier study. The second study was based upon interviews with 81 gang members who were in prison. There is also the problem that the study may have been politically motivated (however sincere the conclusion) and intended at the beginning to produce a counter conclusion to the earlier study. Moreover, the first report was on the role of the gangs in the drug trade, while the second was on the role of drugs in the gangs. The studies did not really research the same question. The difference does not necessarily appear to be of facts but of interpretations of facts.

Furthermore, regarding this latter point, neither study examined, for example, the amount of cocaine the gangs were responsible for bringing into the market compared to an estimate of the total cocaine market in the Los Angeles area (which is not to criticize the studies but rather to point out what was beyond the scope of each). Such a comparison would then give us more of an understanding of how much gangs actually contribute to the problem, not that such data is readily obtained or non-controversial.

We do not know much about how such markets operate. Perhaps gangs are largely responsible at one level (the wholesale) or perhaps they are completely dependent upon larger organized crime groups who import the goods and make the original distribution. Perhaps gangs are largely responsible for the trafficking of drugs in underclass areas, while other networks supply other areas of the city. What is probably true is that dealers observe the same neighborhood (class) boundaries we all observe (which is not to say buyers do). In such a case, where gangs are just the dealers in their neighborhoods, an enforcement policy that stresses busts of underclass gangs will have little effect on the supply side of the market. This is what we would expect to find and this is what we do find. Nonetheless, there is a paucity of research.

Gangs are also expanding beyond their urban centers. Officials estimate that there are very few states without a Los Angeles gang outpost. Violence has not accompanied the gangs, instead, as supply outlets are established for cocaine and "crack," the gang members have gone out of their way to be as inconspicuous as possible. As Kansas City Police Captain David Barton put in, stated in the *New York Times*: "We are not seeing the same kind of gang activity as L.A. When they leave California, they become a drug organization, not a gang."[8]

Furthermore, in a fine example of the paradoxic of behavior, despite the negatives associated with gangs, middle-class and affluent youth are beginning to form gangs of their own patterned after underclass gangs. The media is often blamed for its negative influence upon youth (here as well, for their untiring promotion of alcohol), however, it is difficult to see how the media created such an effect as copying gangs.

Perhaps the very volume of ink and film devoted to the gangs, plus the fear the gangs arouse in the media and, apparently, among police, accounts for the allure. In any event, even as goods gain "mystique" by being forbidden, so too people, or at least condemned adolescents, can gain such "mystique" in the eyes of other adolescents.

Regarding current policy, consider that the continuation of current drug laws plays into the hands of hard-core gangs and would serve to preserve their profits. Current laws gave life to and continue to empower such gangs. Moreover, such "gangs" do not exist and could not exist in a vacuum. They are supported by mainstream financial institutions, middle-class citizens, elected officials and police officials, as well as by the average "dealing as a second job" sort of participant in the underground market.

Such collaboration is nothing new either; this is the traditional history of organized crime. What is different this time is that the faces of gang members are this era's underclass, and that the term "gangs" is used rather than "organized crime." But the fact remains the same. To assure the continued expansion of the gangs, one need only make sure the drug laws remain as they are today.

With the underground market, there not only comes the gangs and the violence associated with them, there also comes the problem of official corruption. As noted in previous chapters, there have been indictments of DEA agents, judges, prosecutors, and mayors. In addition, there is the problem of police officers helping themselves to a share of the drug cash confiscated in raids. In September 1989, some eighteen veterans of a special anti-drug unit of the Los Angeles Sheriff's Department were relieved of duty for allegedly skimming money from their drug busts.[9]

Preliminary estimates were that $200,000 might have been put in their pockets. However, such an estimate must be low, given that vacation homes, power boats, and furniture worth some $300,000 were confiscated by Federal agents from just two deputies.[10] Beyond the immediate problem, complications were created in ongoing drug cases of the special unit, leading to the dismissal of one case and endangering the prosecution of ten others.[11]

Corruption does not stop there; the underground market in drugs produces enormous volumes of cash that must be "laundered" in order to be used for purchases of goods and services (a particular problem in a society that is moving farther and farther away from transactions on a cash basis). Laundering money requires the cooperation of law-abiding citizens and businesses. Ultimately, without such cooperation, the cash would stay cash and be useful only for small item purchases. As there is a law that all bank transactions greater than $10,000 be reported to the IRS, banks are a key agent in money laundering. Banks, and certainly not only banks, upholding the profit motive above community needs (just the same as the gangs), have been very cooperative in helping to launder money.

Caribbean banks have a special reputation for hospitality to money-launderers, but European and American banks also can be found who are more than willing to help out. Moreover, such activities fit into the pre-existing values and practices of some banks, since they provide a haven for those seeking to hide income from the IRS.

The drug trade fits very nicely into pre-existing niches of the market *internationale*. One banker of a French-owned Caribbean bank quoted in *Time* puts it this way (referring to laundering for drug traffickers): "Many of your largest corporations, many of your movie stars, do much the same thing. We wouldn't want to handle criminal money, of course. But if it's just a matter of taxes, that is of no concern to us."[12]

The sums involved are in the billions. In 1985, the Federal Reserve of Miami posted a $6 billion excess. As of 1988 that had fallen to $4.5 billion, but the Los Angeles surplus increased from $116 million to $3.8 billion in 1988 (making for a combined $8.3 billion surplus). There is other evidence of the enormity of the cash flow in illegal transactions, primarily from the drug trade: the U.S. Treasury is unable to account for 80 percent of all currency presently in circulation.

Another effect of the free and immense flow of drug cash is the creation of "upstanding citizen" crime, quite apart from official corruption. In February 1988, Los Angeles police arrested more than 30 suspects, most of them jewelers, who allegedly participated in laundering the proceeds of the cocaine trade. Two "kingpins" were reportedly described as "pleasant, apparently honorable businessmen."[13] "He was just like the 9-to-5 person," one associate stated. "There was nothing suspicious at all."[14] According to the Los Angeles Times report, officials have estimated that the ring had laundered more than one billion dollars worth of drug money.[15]

There are many similar such stories, stories of otherwise respectable citizens participating in laundering and drug-related activities. For example, in Los Angeles, the late UCLA basketball booster and local businessman Sam Gilbert has been said to have derived large profits from money-laundering activities.[16] Even famed baseball player Pete Rose has had his name linked to drug money.[17]

Mr. Bush, commenting upon the L.A. sheriffs accused of skimming money obtained during drug busts, called them "bad apples."[18] However, of the people noted here, seemingly law-abiding (even law enforcing) and otherwise responsible citizens and individuals, none were "evil" per se. Rather, the tremendous amounts of money produced by the underground market proved to be too big a temptation to pass up. Perhaps we should think about our own response, were we given an opportunity to so easily enrich ourselves. Such is the evil of the underground market and it is an evil created not by drugs but by drug laws.

One set of problems associated with the underground market is created by current laws. There is a critical second set: the problems by enforcement itself, meaning the overwhelming of courts and prisons with drug law offenders. According to the former "drug czar," William Bennett, the American people, along with gangs, must be blamed for the failure to mitigate the drug crisis, primarily by refusing to allow the government to build prisons in their neighborhoods.[19] Of course, such new prisons are never proposed for construction in neighborhoods where, for example, top-level government officials and similar professionals live. Instead, such officials propose to build these facilities in the underclass areas of the city.

There are other problems with the prison construction solution as well. Before detailing these problems (most have already been introduced here or will be familiar to the reader), let us look at the problem of a shortage of prison space.

That there is such a problem seems real enough, at least on the surface. On the Federal level, some 46,000 inmates are squeezed into facilities designed to hold 30,000 inmates. The Bush administration has proposed new expenditures of $1.5 billion to expand the Federal prison system. However, according to Justice Department estimates, even if all such expenditures are approved and the prison space built, at the present rate of increased incarceration (which the administration wants more of rather than less) the Federal inmate population will grow to 84,000. This would leave the system short 17,000 beds, even after the expenditure of $1.5 billion.

Moreover, the Bush administration has proposed little help for state and local governments, the governing bodies which must carry the bulk of the burden of fighting drugs and crime. This is a critical point, 42 states are presently under court order to reduce over-crowding. Yet the Bush administration would have these governments arrest and imprison more people even though there is no space for the present population. Further, this is occurring even as many state and local governments are under funding limitations that have led to cutbacks in public safety units such as police, fire, and health departments.

The story of prison overpopulation is remarkably uniform from state to state. In Georgia, the state's prison system can hold 20,000 inmates. Yet, due primarily to increased drug arrests, some 15,000 new prisoners must be housed this year alone. In Los Angeles County, some 22,000 are crowded into facilities designed for 13,000 and more than 100,000 prisoners have been given early release solely to relieve the problem of overcrowding. In New York City, prisoners often sleep on the floor and in rooms in which 90 men must share one toilet. Texas is one state in which William Bennett should be well-pleased; in 1983 the state spent nearly $300 million on prison operations and new construction and in 1988 that figure was increased to $500 million. Yet the system is still so overcrowded that six times in 1989 the state was forced to close its doors to any new inmates. The stories go on and on with little variation.

The question is: what is the point? Overall, even if prison space were doubled nationwide, at a cost estimated to be $43 billion, a criminal's chances of being incarcerated would be no more than one in ten. The system has certainly answered the call for more arrests and more imprisonments; there has been a 161.4 percent jump in drug convictions and a 48.7 percent increase in defendants found guilty of Federal crimes between 1980 and 1987 (the report did not separate to drug-related and non-drug-related crimes).[20] Yet crime is increasing and so is the drug market. The sole result has been to clog an already overloaded prison system. Moreover, not only are prisons overloaded, the entire criminal justice system suffers from such an overload.

The American Bar Association, in a report issued in December 1988, found the justice system to be overwhelmed by the huge but largely unsuccessful effort to deal with the drug crisis via the law enforcement route: "Police, prosecutors and judges told the committee that they have been unsuccessful in making a significant impact on the importation, sale, and use of illegal drugs, despite devoting much of their resources to the arrest, prosecution and trial of drug offenders."[21] The Los Angeles Times reports from the same source: "These extraordinary efforts have instead distorted and overwhelmed the criminal justice system, crowding dockets and jails, and diluting law enforcement and judicial efforts to deal with other major criminal cases."[22]

Yet Federal officials overlook such inconvenient expert testimony and continue to insist upon more arrests and more jails. In California, the state Judicial Council estimates that 60 to 65 percent of all cases in court are now drug-related. "In some courts, they [drug-related cases] are pushing civil cases out almost entirely," Judge Richard P. Byrne, presiding judge of Los Angeles Superior Court has been quoted as stating.[23]

"This is a societal problem," Judge Byrne has said. "More arrests...and more prosecutions aren't going to solve it.... To the extent we can, we need more education, treatment, and the acceptance of personal responsibility. We can't abandon enforcement— I'm very much opposed to legalization—but we do have to take a broader approach to the problem."[24]

There is yet another point. Before the latest push to imprison yet more individuals, we were already one of the world's leaders in number of people imprisoned as a percentage of total population. Only South Africa and the Soviet Union surpassed America in percentage of citizens behind bars. Today, as an outcome of the "war against drugs," we have outdone those two countries and the United States now leads the world in numbers of citizens in jail per capita. Do we really want such a dubious distinction? Does such a distinction speak well for American democracy?

Moreover, there is a particular sort of citizen being arrested and jailed: members of the underclass. And there is a particular sort of citizen not being arrested and not going to jail: members of the middle and upper classes. Eighty percent of non-mainstream drug users are white (the proportion of whites in the general population). However, as Chicago Judge Thomas Sumner was quoted as stating: "Judging by what I see, I would have thought the numbers would be totally reversed."[25]

"There's as much cocaine in the Sears Tower or in the stock exchange as there is in the black community," Charles Ramsey, commander of the Chicago police department's narcotics division is quoted as stating. "But those guys are harder to catch. Those deals are done in office buildings, in somebody's home, and there's not the violence associated with it that there is in the black community. But the guy standing on the corner, he's almost got a sign on his back. These guys are just arrestable."[26]

"One of the problems is you get a community demanding numbers," Assistant U.S. Attorney Tim Discenza is quoted as stating. "So, if you are an elected mayor or sheriff or other elected official, you may want to use officers in long-term arrests of suppliers that, after three months, may only result in two people being arrested. On the other hand, you can use those same officers and make 200 arrests."[27]

So the problem is larger than the police. Given the current hysteria, the demand is for higher arrest figures and police officials are bound to comply, even in cases where it might be against their better judgement. The outcome is paid for by the underclass and without any substantial reduction in demand or supply. The result: in the United States 25 percent of African-American males in their twenties are under court supervision (compared to some 6 percent of white males of the same age). Overall, the United States now imprisons four times more members of the black male population (per capita) than South Africa. The figures are as follows: 3,000 per 100,000 African American males are imprisoned compared to 700 per 100,000 South African black males.

In summary, the first set of problems associated with the current policy originates in the construction of an underground market. The second set of problems comes from drug law enforcement, the outcome of which is the overcrowding of the courts and prisons. This leads us to the third set of problems associated with the law enforcement approach: the problem of the expansion of governmental and police power. What follows is a presentation of various measures passed in recent years as part of the "war against drugs."

Within the law enforcement community there have been a steady stream of proposals and actions from law and policymakers. Under a 1984 law, police are empowered to confiscate property purchased with drug money. In 1987, some 9,129 properties worth $480 million had been seized; in 1988 the figures increased to 16,150 properties with a value of $704 million.[28] In order to keep the property, police must show only a "preponderance of evidence" that drug money was used to purchase the object or property, a lower standard than the usual criminal proof of beyond a reasonable doubt. Only 10 percent of such cases are contested in court.[29]

The benefits of the policy, on its own terms, is that it gives local departments an incentive to focus on drug cases, particularly during a time of civic budget crunches. One risk of such a policy is that it encourages departments to work on their own and not cooperate with other police agencies, for to call upon another department means sharing the spoils.

The funds involved are not small. For example, since 1985, the LAPD has seized funds and assets worth over $100 million.[30] According to police officials (of course, such officials are not disinterested spectators), competition between departments has been known to destroy a case, but this is said to be a rare exception.

Of course, there are other problems with such a policy. It encourages police to place a higher priority on drug cases than on all other cases. Furthermore, it encourages the police to violate civil liberties in their zeal to get the loot. However, concern with constitutional liberties and the balance between individual liberty and government empowerment is not a great concern in the general hysteria of government policymakers.

The U.S. Supreme Court has upheld the power of the government to seize the money and assets of drug defendants even if such seizure means the defendants are unable to hire an attorney for their defense.[31] According to Justice Byron White, writing in favor of the law, even as a bank robber may not claim he has a right to keep some of the money to pay an attorney, so too a drug dealer should not be allowed to use drug money to hire an attorney. Justice Harry A. Blackmun wrote in dissent: "It is unseemly and unjust for the government to beggar those it prosecutes in order to disable their defense at trial."[32] The vote on the issue before the Court was 5-4 in favor. The president of the National Association of Criminal Defense Attorneys, Ephraim Margolin, reacted this way: "The Supreme Court by a margin of one simply felt that the right to counsel of choice can be done away with."[33]

A second dissenting opinion came from the attorney that defended John DeLorean in his celebrated drug case: "It presumes guilt," according to Los Angeles defense attorney Harry Weitzman. "It also gives the government an additional power in criminal prosecutions that they just should not have."[34]

The ruling in question was on all illegally obtained funds, including, for example, gains from money laundering or insider stock trading. However, law authorities have not used the law against Wall Street brokers accused of insider trading or against savings and loans executives accused of looting the public: the law has only been applied to drug cases. This is another example of uneven enforcement; the government was reluctant to act against Shell and Exxon's supplying of the underground market with the chemicals needed to make cocaine—even as the government takes action against mom and pop-type suppliers of horticultural equipment.

The expansion of the power of the Federal government goes further; the U.S. government has handed itself the power to make arrests on foreign territory. Of course, the White House administration has the power to hand itself that power since constitutional restrictions stop at the border. However, where constitutional restrictions end, international conventions begin and there is no doubt that attempts to enforce such a self-granted power would raise an uproar in the affected country. Mr. Bush has stated that he was unaware that such a power existed.[35]

Congress too has adopted the law enforcement approach. In September 1988, the House made it a death penalty offense when murders are committed in the course of a violation of Federal drug laws.[36] And judges are passing tougher sentences. A Federal judge in Los Angeles sentenced a 22-year-old man to life in prison without parole for possession of 5.5 ounces of crack, a rather small amount in terms of the thriving drug market (probably a two or three day supply for an individual user). The judge declared:

"Congress has gone out to battle the drug war and this man is one of the enemies."[37]

Extreme sentences may be self-defeating. Such sentencing may deter some but may also encourage violence in others by raising the stakes for capture. Hence, such sentencing may lead to an escalation of violence rather than a diminution. What is possible is that there will be a winnowing out of dealers, with deterrence working to keep casual dealers out of the field only to leave the market in the hands of career criminals unfazed by such consequences. Moreover, there are violent offenders who are going to be released back to the streets to make way for the increase in drug law offenders placed behind bars.

There is the further problem of exploiting laws initially intended to address a specific part of the drug problem and using those laws as broadly as possible. Further there remains, as always, the problem of uneven enforcement. Congress passed a measure that most people could support, a law that made it a Federal offense to sell drugs within 1,000 feet of a schoolyard or 100 feet of a playground or video arcade.[38]

Unfortunately, there is a problem with how that law is being enforced. In Los Angeles, of 92 people charged under the new law, 91 have been African American or Hispanic. Police claimed they go where the problem is greatest, but, of course, there are "white" schools with just as much of a problem in drug dealing as underclass schools. An assistant U.S. attorney, speaking in defense of the skewed arrests, stated he did not know that there was a problem for, he said: "We don't keep records on race."[39]

There is the problem of the expansion and distortion of the original intent of the law. The law was originally meant to be used against individuals who were selling to youngsters in school; however, it is being used against individuals who live within the given radius even if no school dealing is involved.

For example, a twenty-year-old woman was charged and convicted under the new law after selling $25 worth of crack to an elderly LAPD informant in her boyfriend's apartment. The apartment was in a housing project within 1,000 feet of a schoolyard. She received a five-year mandated sentence. Some federal judges are reported to have expressed reservations about such use of the law (and, once again, an underclass neighborhood was involved, not a middle- or upper-middle-class neighborhood).

However much the sale of crack can be condemned, there is the further problem of the continued expansion of police power. Once authorities are granted such special powers, originally intended for a specific application to a specific problem, the powers granted are used in a way that police authorities find most convenient in their work, quite apart from the original intention of lawmakers. In this way, the expansion of police authority, and the resulting threat to individual liberty, takes on a certain life of its own.[40]

The House also passed legislation that would overturn the so-called exclusionary rule in drug cases.[41] The exclusionary rule prevents the admission in court of evidence that is illegally obtained by police. The new yardstick would be that the evidence could be used so long as it was obtained by police in "good-faith" that their actions did not violate the Fourth Amendment prohibiting illegal searches and seizures. Critics maintain this standard is a practical impossibility and, in effect, overturns the Fourth Amendment. Charles Rangel of New York argued that this loosening of constitutional protection meant "...the war on drugs is becoming a war on the Constitution."[42]

In the most recent test of the constitutionality of the relaxation of Fourth Amendment protections, the California State Supreme Court and the U.S. Supreme Court supported the traditional interpretation of the exclusionary rule. The Attorney General of California had first asked the State Supreme Court and then the U.S. Supreme Court to overturn a lower court's opinion that favored the older and stricter interpretation of the exclusionary rule. Both Courts refused to hear the case, in effect ratifying the traditional standard of search and seizure.[43]

Nonetheless, in other cases the Court has approved the whittling down of search and seizure protections. For example, the Court has upheld the use of drug courier profiles as a basis for stopping and questioning individuals.[44] This has proven to be a particular problem for well-dressed African-American males. The Court has also upheld the searching of automobiles without a search warrant and the obtaining of a search warrant based on an anonymous informant's tip, among other such exceptions to traditional protections.

The House also passed other anti-drug laws that day. Veterans convicted of drug distribution would lose benefits such as housing loans and education. Students convicted of drug crimes would lose their student loans.[45] In addition, all students receiving Pell Grant Student Aid are required to sign a statement stating they "...will not engage in the unlawful manufacture, distribution, dispensation, possession or use of a controlled substance."[46]

Families in public housing could be evicted from their homes if a member of the family were convicted of a drug offense.[47] This is an echo of a recent California law, a statute that allows police to arrest any parents who have, in the opinion of police, failed their parental duties by allowing their children to participate in a street gang.[48]

The first such arrest under this California law was made in April 1989. The mother arrested said the investigation made by police amounted to one phone call to her and during that call it was never stated that she was under investigation. The mother's (this was a single parent household) 15-year-old son had been previously arrested by police for a number of serious crimes. Her response was to enroll herself in a parental education and counseling program and to place her son in an alternative education school.[49] The police, after first claiming the mother was "actively involved in her son's gang," withdrew charges ten days later.[50]

Washington policymakers not only argue for the expansion of federal and local police power, they urge state governments to follow suit. In May 1989, former drug czar William J. Bennett proposed a "model" legislative package for state governments that would, he claimed, significantly mitigate the drug crisis.[51] The measures he advocated would mandate weekend incarceration of first-time offenders, give authority to local police to suspend and revoke the driver's license of individuals arrested for drug offenses, allow confiscation of their automobiles, and severely fine and even imprison parents of individuals convicted of drug offenses. According to Bennett, parents "...must bear responsibility for the behavior and activities of minors in their charge."[52] Even, apparently, when incarcerated in jail for their failure to do so.

But this is not enough, according to Bennett. Comparing the current crisis to the Civil War, Bennett has argued before Congress that even as Lincoln saw fit to suspend habeas corpus during the Civil War, so too we should consider limiting this traditionally sacrosanct constitutional right in order to win this war on drugs. "This war is not for delicate sensibilities," Bennett argued in April 1989. "This is tough stuff."[53] The right of habeas corpus is the constitutional right of a citizen to know what they were arrested for and requires the police to prove that a crime was in fact committed.

The Bush administration would not stop there. Mr. Bennett argued that the military should be empowered to arrest civilians and to otherwise assume police duties. Mr. Bennett went on to state that his mind was open to other possibilities of expanding the government's power to fight the drug war. The overall impact of Mr. Bennett's testimony was to lead one senator, Joseph Biden (D-Del), to wonder, "...whether or not you are an ideologue who will reach the conclusion that the ends justify the means as it relates to constitutional protections."[54]

Given the problems associated with the law enforcement approach, what has been the response of elected officials? More of the same—including bringing in the military. A number of members of Congress have actively supported the use of the military in the drug crisis. Indeed, there is a certain consensus in the Congress and the administration that the military should do its share. This led (in 1981) to the repeal of the Posse Comitas Act of 1878, a century old act that forbade the use of the military in civilian affairs.[55]

Former Defense Secretary Frank Carlucci was not enthusiastic about involving the military. His concern was that troops are trained to overcome what is in their path while police enforcement requires sensibility to constitutional protections and, therefore, troops are inappropriate tools of law enforcement. "Our military is not trained to read people their Miranda rights," Carlucci reported to Congress. "They're trained to shoot to kill."[56] Further, an article in *Science* quotes him as stating: "The defense budget is not a slush fund for drug enforcement."[57] Over his objections, Congress ordered the use of AWAC surveillance planes to track air movement over the southern border.[58]

Present Secretary Dick Cheney is taking the opposite tack, announcing in September 1989 that drugs represent "...a direct threat to the sovereignty and security of the country."[59] He added that the U.S. military is now an "enthusiastic participant" in the anti-drug effort. Cheney stated that the military would provide temporary jail space to ease overcrowding and would send military trainers and advisors to Colombia, Peru, and Bolivia to help those countries in their war against drug producers.[60]

This could lead to an interesting scenario. Israeli military advisors who are experts in anti-terrorism have been working with the private armies of the Medellin cocaine cartel of Colombia. The training of the cocaine troops by the Israelis included the how-to's of assaulting a town, ambushing automobiles, and countering such ambushes. The training also included drive-by attacks from moving automobiles and such routine military work as constructing and setting off bombs, as well as ordinary physical training and practices such as obstacle courses and rappelling down hillsides. The Israeli advisors do not deny their involvement, claiming the Colombian government knew of their work and that their training was carried out within sight of a Colombian army base.[61]

The Bush administration, to my knowledge, has not responded to these reports. This could lead to an interesting scenario. Perhaps someday American-trained government troops will fight Israeli-trained cartel troops, and then we can gauge the effectiveness of our military trainers versus the effectiveness of Israeli military trainers. Perhaps we will discover that we have called in the wrong military, that we should have called upon the Israeli military instead of our own! Nonetheless, the military is now on board, their enthusiasm having been given an unexpected boost by the dramatic changes in Eastern Europe. "With peace breaking out all over," one general was quoted as stating. "It might give us something to do."[62]

The Army has proposed stationing troops along the Mexican-American border to track down "mules." The Air Force has proposed, in addition to the AWAC's that are already being used, to send up high-resolution spy satellites to pick out hidden drug laboratories and, in an effort to keep track of movements of drug shipments, to reproduce the high-priced radar system that monitors Warsaw Pact troops.

The Navy, for its part, is offering to place 90 aircraft and 12 ships in the Caribbean. As one retired senior officer, Rear Admiral Eugene Carroll, deputy director of the Washington-based Center for Defense Information, stated: "Drug interdiction is at least a raft to keep you afloat."[63]

The law enforcement option is rapidly developing its own bureaucracy and adding the support of others with a stake in keeping this option the first and foremost response to the drug crisis. Furthermore, the war mentality evident in the "war against drugs," the "anything goes" attitude, entangled as it is in the older social reality of prejudice against the underclass, has a very specific effect at the street level—the problem of police overreaction.

An example of this is the Dalton Ave. police raid in South-Central Los Angeles in the summer of 1988. Some 80 LAPD police officers took part in a nighttime raid on four apartments thought to be "havens" for drug and gang activity. Some 33 people were taken into police custody, six were booked, the others were photographed and released. Of the six that were booked, only one was successfully prosecuted and he was a passerby who did not live in the apartments.[64] More LAPD officers were eventually charged than gang members. But then no gang members were arrested or even found. Out of the 80 officers, 38 were disciplined for their conduct during the raid and of those, 9 were singled out for special investigation.

Some 40 residents filed complaints against the police. They charged that officers had knocked holes in apartment walls, poured bleach on clothing, emptied the contents of refrigerators and freezers upon the floor, spray-painted "LAPD Rules" upon the walls and, in a final bit of pathological behavior, beat, and arrested people who were passersby.[65]

The Red Cross visited the scene and gave the sort of assistance usually reserved for natural disasters. The apartments were judged to be "uninhabitable." The first officer placed before a special investigatory board was found innocent of the serious charges and given two days off without pay. This officer stated, regarding the verdict, that "justice had been served."[66] Four officers were eventually arrested for their actions. One officer pleaded no contest and became a prosecution witness in the trial of the other three. However, all three were found not guilty, jury members telling the press that there was no evidence these three officers in particular were responsible for any of the damage to the apartments.[67] No officer was charged in the beatings. The city of Los Angeles eventually paid out $3 million in restitution and punitive damages to the residents of the apartments.

Beyond the evident loss of perspective on the part of police, there is the continuing feature of underclass neighborhoods being subjected to police actions that would certainly be out-of-bounds in any other kind of neighborhood. Levels of police violence and legal actions are of one sort in underclass neighborhoods, of yet another in middle-class areas. Indeed, one reason there has been no outcry over the whittling down of constitutional protections is that such diminution has been confined to the underclass. The middle class has gotten a more or less free ride regarding the new powers granted police agencies.

What is happening here is that the "war against drugs" has become submerged within far older and larger American social forces and facts: the inability of America (unlike the rest of the developed world) to solve the problem of American poverty and the preference for a law enforcement rather than social welfare approach to poverty. The current policy regarding drugs is a mirror image of the larger policy toward poverty. But more law enforcement can only imprison more poor people without solving any of the problems of drugs or crime or poverty.

This is not to excuse the behavior or crime of any individual. Finally, a society does not make sense, cannot be a society, without individual responsibility. Nonetheless, even as in economics we take a step back from the individual level and thereby interpret the economy and take action on the basis of a structural analysis rather than on the basis of "individual responsibility," so too we need to apply a structural perspective to American society if we are to get at the roots of the lack of social peace. The Dalton Ave. raid cannot be understood solely on the basis of the actions of the particular individuals who took part in the raid. What happened on Dalton Ave. must also be understood as one episode of a too-old and too-familiar story.

One might simply claim racism on the part of the Los Angeles Police Department, or say that this department has a particular problem with violence. After all, we have from the same department the example of the Rodney King beating and the fact that Los Angeles paid out over $11 million in 1990 to resolve police abuse charges.[68] However, given the national statistics regarding the incarceration rates of African American males, the evidence is that the problem goes beyond any one department.

This is not to excuse or overlook the particular problems of a particular department. Rather, it makes sense to try to understand how racism, an evil few if any of us evade, was made possible here. In other words, what disinhibited the police and permitted their racism to surface in a way that was imperceptible to many (probably not all) of the individuals involved? How can this be explained?

Herbert J. Gans, in a classic work of urban sociology, *The Urban Villagers*, categorized the people of underclass neighborhoods as being of two sorts: the majority were people who held middle-class values, meaning they cared for their children and valued education but did not have middle-class incomes. These he called the "urban villagers." There was a second group, the violent and lost element he called the "urban jungle." The difficulty for police (and for the majority of the residents of these neighborhoods) is that both groups share the same streets and buildings. Nor is an outsider likely to tell by appearance alone of which group a particular individual is a member.

No doubt the intention of the LAPD was to take action against the members of the urban jungle. However, it was the members of the urban village, living a settled and relatively stable life, that were the victims of the raid and are, unless adequate precautions are taken, bound to be the victims again—simply because they are the residents that can be found. The members of the urban jungle are considerably more elusive. Still, the urban villagers, given their values, could well be the allies of police against gangs and crime. Yet this is hardly possible if the police lump all residents of underclass neighborhoods together in one negative category.

One example of the middle-class orientation of the villagers comes from a recent story in the *Los Angeles Times*. A mother, after becoming aware that her son was wanted by the police in connection with a shooting, called the police and promised to bring her teenage son into custody the next day. The sergeant on duty recalled his skepticism. Nonetheless, the next day, as promised, the mother brought in her son.

Both attitudes are typical; the middle-class orientation of the mother and the ignorance of the police that such an attitude is common in such neighborhoods.

As regards social policy, the existence of the urban villagers is promising. In terms of immediate action, here is a resource for the police. In terms of long-term action, these are the people willing to help themselves. Yet, whenever the needs of such neighborhoods are raised, the response is that there is not the money to provide more services. There is money, however, for increased police action, such as the yearly Federal increases for more law enforcement. But such action misses the mark, does little more than feed the public bias and leaves the underlying conditions, and the underlying potential for positive change, untouched.

What more might help? Current thinking is more technology. The military's anti-smuggling effort is a combined service effort based in southern Florida and in California. These units use AWAC planes and Navy combat ships to detect air and sea movements that are in some way suspicious. More high-tech military solutions are on the way. Moreover, this could be just the beginning of the application of technology to the anti-drug effort.

Los Alamos researchers (the place where the nuclear bomb was invented and where nuclear research continues) are also becoming involved. Physicists have proposed lasers that would detect fumes from jungle drug-making laboratories. Biologists have proposed sophisticated bacteria that would remove the psychoactive effect of the coca leaf. Others propose isotope fertilizers that would make illicit crops radioactive, stun guns that would disable engines, as well as the application of supercomputers that would track the drug shipments of the underground market. How the latter option might work is beyond this author's knowledge and perhaps, the proponents.

There are, however, simpler solutions in place, solutions, that are perfectly compatible with the law enforcement approach but for which no new funding is proposed by Washington policymakers. These are solutions with a human touch and a human face that offer, in addition to law enforcement, simple hope. In short, there are the Officer Kilroys of the country, as mentioned in a story that appeared in the *Los Angeles Times*.

Officer Howard Kilroy is a Chicago policeman who for 17 years has kept tabs on a Chicago schoolyard and kept it free of the drug dealers and violence that have become, in many neighborhoods, an accepted part of the meaning of "going to school." The underclass neighborhood in which the Kosciuszko elementary school of Chicago is located is plagued with these kinds of problems. But not the schoolyard, due to Officer Kilroy's efforts.[69] He has earned the respect and affection of every child, parent and teacher of the school. He has been described as "...a throwback to a bygone era when cops walked beats, knew everybody by name and were seen by children as role models, not objects of hate or fear."[70]

Officer Kilroy insists he is not special. Speaking of the children, he states: "They're just starving for someone, anyone, to look up to...I've always liked kids. I just think it's our job to win friends. We have enough enemies already."[71] But the people who know of Kilroy's work tell another story. He is described as "...a genuinely nice, unpretentious guy who walks kids home from school, sponsors neighborhood ball teams with money from his own pocket and stands in for Santa Claus at the school Christmas pageant."[72]

The assistant principal of the school tells of gang fights he has broken up by his very presence. "People that don't even speak English know him well," states Emma Lozano, president of the community parent-teacher council. "They respect him and feel comfortable with him around their children. He's become sort of an institution around here."[73]

What made this story a national one was that Kilroy got transferred. It was the familiar story of a hard-pressed police department that decided to switch officers off foot patrol to squad cars, expanding the range that an understaffed police force can patrol. But the resulting uproar from the neighborhood and school was so great that Kilroy's transfer was reversed and he is now back at Kosciuszko school.

One suspects there are other Officer Kilroys out there in the country, and there could be more if this solution to this aspect of the drug crisis was given a try. Moreover, what could be a more obvious solution to the problem of drugs and violence in the schoolyard than to station an officer in these schoolyards? And in making the schoolyard a regular beat for individual officers, so they can become known and trusted by the neighborhood and school. Of course, such a person would have to appreciate and find worthwhile the special nature of working with very young people.

Naturally, it would require funding to pay for such solutions. But the Federal government alone is spending $8 billion a year on drug law enforcement without any evidence that this spending is effective. For a fraction of that $8 billion worth of high-tech law enforcement, dedicated and effective officers such as Howard Kilroy could be found for every schoolyard.

To summarize, drug laws create an underground market. With this market, there comes the problems of police and official corruption, as well as the problem of "honest citizen" and "upstanding citizen" type crime. Another critical problem generated by such an underground market is the empowerment of professional and violent offenders undeterred by the possibility of prison time. The chief effect of law enforcement may be to winnow out the weaker competitors, thereby clearing the field for the more experienced and dangerous.

Underground markets are produced and maintained by current law, and then enforcement efforts bring their own distinctive problems. Public opinion has not been unheard; more arrests, more convictions, more people sent to jail, all this and more is being done. But the unintended consequence of so simplistically meeting the public demand has been the early release of violent offenders so that space can be cleared for drug offenders. The streets are no safer than before.

At the level of policymaking, there is the problem of the expansion of governmental power. Historically, once a government expands its power over the lives of individuals, it does not give up such authority readily. Nor are governments reluctant to expand beyond constitutional protections: "Throughout [American] history, the government has said we're in an unprecedented crisis and that we must live without civil liberties until the crisis is over," Yale Kamisar of the University of Michigan School of Law is quoted as stating. "It's a hoax."[74]

Milton Friedman, leading conservative and a Nobel Prize-winning economist, wrote an open letter to former drug czar William Bennett in September 1989: "The path you propose of more police, more jails, use of the military in foreign countries, harsh penalties for drug users, and a whole panoply of repressive measures can only make a bad situation worse. The drug war cannot be won with those tactics without undermining the human liberty and individual freedom that you and I cherish."[75]

The outcome of such policies has been a law enforcement effort that has run amok. A war mentality has been encouraged in which no solution is ignored, however repressive, however counter to the best of American history and tradition. Moreover, the failure of such policies has only led to calls for more of the same. This is a textbook example of a public hysteria.

Furthermore, the reluctance of many to challenge the hysteria, the clear ground provided the most negative of proponents, combined with the compliance of media reporters who unthinkingly repeat the worst possible interpretations is how the hysteria is maintained. Public and political anxieties feed off one another, with the news media the conduit by which this is done. Rather than countering popular prejudice with studied opinion, most news stories reflect back existing social biases as fact, and so the hysteria is fueled rather than extinguished.

There are genuine concerns. There is a genuine core of truth in the problem of illegal usage. However, the mindlessness of the response to these genuine problems and the heedlessness of the consequences of such a response, these are the signs of a hysteria. The picture is completed when we find public officials such as Mayor Kurt Schmoke of Baltimore, officials who honestly relate the problems of the current approach, becoming targets of anger. Others become yet more reluctant to speak out against the blindness of popular policy. Hence the policy continues unabated, even as evidence of failure and unintended consequences continues to build.

Notes

1. "Talent for the Drug Game: Tough and Loyal Athletes Recruited by Cocaine Rings," *Los Angeles Times,* 28 November 1988, II 1:1.
2. "Esther Crighton Has Respect: A 12-year-old Fulfills His Mother's Dreams With Drug Profits," *Los Angeles Times,* 10 September 1989, V 5:1.
3. Peter Reuter, et al., *Money from Crime: A Study of the Economics of Drug Dealing in Washington D.C.,* R-3894-RF (Santa Monica: RAND Corporation, 1990).
4. Ibid., ix.
5. "Black Gangs' Role in Drug Trade Overblown, Study Finds," *Los Angeles Times,* 8 September 1988, II 1:1.
6. "Study Tightly Links Gangs to Trafficking in Cocaine," *Los Angeles Times,* 15 November 1989, B 2:3.
7. Ibid.
8. "Armed, Sophisticated and Violent, Two Drug Gangs Blanket Nation," New York Times, 25 November 1988, I 14.
9. "Drug Funds Missing, 9 Deputies Suspended," *Los Angeles Times,* 2 September 1989, I 1:2.
10. "U.S. Seizes Property of Suspended Deputies," *Los Angeles Times,* 26 September 1989, I 1:3.
11. "Deputies Role Leads to Dismissal of Drug Case," *Los Angeles Times,* 27 September 1989, I 1:1.
12. " A Torrent of Dirty Dollars," *Time,* 18 December 1989, 50.
13. "Solid Gold Shock," *Los Angeles Times,* 24 February 1989, II 1:1.
14. Ibid.
15. Ibid.
16. "Miami Trial Gives Startling New Portrait of Sam Gilbert," *Los Angeles Times,* 23 April 1990, A 25:2.
17. "Rose Wanted Part of Drug Ring, Janzen Says," *Los Angeles Times,* 28 June 1990, D 1:1.
18. "President Seeks to Reassure L.A. Deputy Sheriffs," *Los Angeles Times,* 2 March 1990, A 1:5.
19. "Don't Resist New Prisons, Bennett Pleads," *Los Angeles Times,* 20 October 1989, A 22:1.
20. A number of articles are relevant here including "New Tactics in the War on Drugs Tilt Scales of Justice Off-Balance," New York Times, 29 December 1989, I 1:1; "California Leads U.S. in Inmate Increase," *Los Angeles Times,* 21 May 1990, A 3:2; "Our Bulging Prisons," *Time,* 29 May 1989, 28-31.
21. Quoted in "Drug Cases Clog Justice System ABA Concludes," *Los Angeles Times,* 1 December 1988, I 1:1.
22. Ibid.
23. "Drug Cases Now Dominate Caseloads of Urban Courts," *Los Angeles Times,* 23 April 1990, A 24.
24. Ibid.
25. "Black Feel Brunt of Drug War." *Los Angeles Times,* 22 April 1990, A 26.
26. Ibid., A 1.

27. Ibid., A 26.
28. "Seizures of Real Estate Stepped Up in War on Drugs," *Los Angeles Times*, 6 November 1988, I 1:1.
29. "Police Departments Enjoy a Boom From Their Drug Busts," *Los Angeles Times*, 23 October 1988, II 1:4.
30. "Depriving Drug Suspects of Lawyers Fees Ok'd," *Los Angeles Times*, 23 June 1989, A 30.
31. Ibid.
32. Ibid.
33. "Lawyers Critical of Rulings on Seizure of Attorney Fees," *Los Angeles Times*, 23 June 1989, A 20.
34. Ibid.
35. "Ruling Backs U.S. Forces Police Role," *Los Angeles Times*, 17 December 1989, A 1:4.
36. "House Votes Death For Drug Murders," New York Times, 9 September 1988, I 1:1.
37. "5 1/2 ounces of Crack Brings Life Term With No Parole," *Los Angeles Times*, 7 December 1989, A36:1. Both the defendant and the judge were African Americans.
38. "Judges Probe Prosecutors Choices on Drug Arrests," *Los Angeles Times*, 14 November 1989, B 1:5.
39. Ibid., B4.
40. Regarding selective enforcement, another story focused on schoolyards and the claim that minority schools received a disproportionate amount of police attention. One such article is "Schoolyard Drug Law Bias Charge to be Probed," *Los Angeles Times*, 13 November 1989, B 1:5.
41. "House Votes Death For Drug Murders," New York Times, 9 September 1988, I 1:4.
42. Ibid., I 1.
43. "Exclusionary Rule Appeal Refused by High Court," *Los Angeles Times*, 31 May 1989. The case referred to is Leichty v. California 88-1666, I 3:5.
44. Florida v. Royer, 460 U.S. 491, 493 (1983). U.S. v. Montoya (1985).
45. "House Votes Death For Drug Murders," New York Times, 9 September 1988, I 1:4.
46. "Anti-Drug Statement Added For Pell Grant," *Daily Nexus*, 2 June 1989. This is the student newspaper of the University of California at Santa Barbara.
47. "House Votes Death For Drug Murders," New York Times, 9 September 1988, I 1:4.
48. "Mother Seized Under Gang Law Cleared," *Los Angeles Times*, 10 June 1989, I 1:3.
49. "Mother Arrested Under Gang Law Denies Blame," *Los Angeles Times*, 31 May 1989, I 1:1.
50. Ibid.
51. "Bennett Outlines Anti-Drug Plan," *Los Angeles Times*, 4 May 1989, I 1:5.
52. Ibid.

53. "Bennett Would Limit Rights in War on Drugs," *Los Angeles Times*, 3 March 1989, I 1:2.
54. Ibid., I20.
55. Eliot Marshall, "A War on Drugs With Real Troops?" *Science* 240 (July 1988): 13-15.
56. "In Reversal, Military Seeks Drug War Role," *Los Angeles Times*, 15 December 1989, A 1:4.
57. Ibid., A 13.
58. "In Reversal, Military Seeks Drug War Role," *Los Angeles Times*, 15 December 1989, A 1:4.
59. "Wider Anti-Drug Role Announced For Pentagon," *Los Angeles Times*, 19 September 1989, I 6:1.
60. Ibid.
61. "Tape Shows Israelis Training Cartel's Killers," *Los Angeles Times*, 30 August 1989, I 1:2.
62. "In Reversal, Military Seeks Drug War Role," *Los Angeles Times*, 15 December 1989, A 36.
63. Ibid.
64. "U.S. Probing Police Raid On Apartments," *Los Angeles Times*, 2 September 1989, I 1:3.
65. Ibid.
66. "Officer Absolved of Most Charges in Massive Raid," *Los Angeles Times*, 26 August 1989, D4. Moreover, an example can be found of police action that, in an effort to contain the drug trade, actively abetted and aided the trade in an underclass neighborhood ("Did Cocaine Sting Fuel Drug Sales?" *Los Angeles Times*, 14 June 1989). The story comes from Cleveland and is a rather complicated one. In essence, police were offered a rare opportunity to work with a large-scale drug dealer, through the dealer get to a major Colombian distributor and, or so local authorities initially hoped, even to the source of the cocaine in Colombia. Going to Colombia became out of the question because of DEA objections but the sting of the Colombian distributor became a live case.

The police allowed the dealer to open a drug house that operated in Cleveland's underclass neighborhood 7 days a week, 12 hours a day. The dealer told employees not to worry, that the police were protecting the house. Indeed, in approximately three months time the dealer was able to pile up some $500,000 in profits. The profits were stored in brown paper bags and kept in a secure place, a safe in the police chief's office. Eventually, the money disappeared back into the drug world; it was used to pay off the debts the police informer owed the distributor. However, the Colombian was arrested along with 15 others (6 were convicted and the Colombian sentenced to 15 years in jail) and some 46 kilos of cocaine with an estimated street value of 50 million dollars were confiscated.

The bust was a howling success for the special anti-drug team that organized the sting. However, several months of drug dealing occurred under the protection of the police. Police claimed they did not know where the $500,000 came from and in turn arrested the drug dealer. Several investigations have indicated that police officers must have known the dealer was getting the money from the sale of drugs, including evidence that officers involved in the case warned other units to stay away from the neighborhood where the drug house did its business. Indeed, no one seriously disputes that the police knew of and abetted the sales. However, when the matter went to trial, the judge threw out the case on the grounds that even if the police department knew of the sales and assisted the sales, the sales would be legal (given Ohio laws) for they were performed for a law enforcement purpose.

Residents of the neighborhood were outraged at the police assistance of drug sales in their community. U.S. Representative Louis Stokes has criticized the sales on the grounds, "No decision like this could've been made to have this type of operation on the West Side of Cleveland or anywhere that's predominantly white" (p. 18).

However, Safety Director Mitchell J. Brown, himself African American, states: "First of all, this man was selling drugs since 1972 to the best of our knowledge and the black community never turned his ass in" (p. 19).

This is similar to the thinking that had the CIA assisting the heroin pipeline into the U.S. during the Vietnam War, and had George Bush and Oliver North looking the other way so long as drug traffickers assisted the Contra effort. The thinking of local police officials, evidently, was that the drugs were going to get sold and used anyway so why not use the dealer for their own purposes? However, a prosecutor testified that the special drug squad must have been more concerned with making the front page than in getting drugs off the street, as a sale of 31 ounces is enough to earn a dealer the maximum sentence, but police urged the dealer working with them to set up a 50 kilo deal.

67. "L.A. Officer Charged in Raid Pleads No Contest," *Los Angeles Times*, 23 March 1991, B 1:1

68. "$11.3 Million Paid in 1990 to Resolve Police Abuse Cases," *Los Angeles Times*, 29 March 1991, A 3:1.

69. "Kilroy Is There and Students Hope He'll Stay," *Los Angeles Times*, 9 December 1989, A 1:1.

70. Ibid., A 26.

71. Ibid.

72. Ibid.

73. Ibid.

74. "Uncivil Liberties?" Newsweek, 23 April 1990, 18.

75. Milton Friedman, "An Open Letter to Bill Bennett," *Wall Street Journal*, 7 September 1989, A 14:3.

8

Successful Solutions and

Failed Attempts

American society is a medicine society, a society of members who routinely use drugs of all sorts to maintain and enhance lifestyle. "Drugs," often considered peripheral, are in fact within the very core of the culture, meaning, involved in everyday life and routine interaction with others. Given such a society we would expect to find the problem of abuse and we do. Due to societal ambiguity, inconsistencies abound in society's response to and methods of dealing with the drug crisis.

The question is: what are the alternatives? One alternative is either legalization or decriminalization. Decriminalization means a substance cannot be legally sold, but there is no penalty for possession; legalization means a substance is legal to sell as well as to possess. Legalization—more accurately, exchanging the deregulation of the underground market for aboveground regulation—has been proposed by some experts as a more effective form of social control; a paradoxical form no doubt, but then the current approach itself has the paradoxical effect of producing and rewarding criminal activity via the profits of the underground market.

Furthermore, this is not the first drug crisis through which this country has suffered. Though much of the story of Prohibition is well-known through relentless popularization in books, films, and television, still, to be thorough, it makes sense to at least touch on this era and consider how historians analyze Prohibition. In addition, the cocaine fad of the 1890s will be considered, as well as the narcotics problem that existed at the turn of the century in

Victorian America. What stopped these crises? We should be aware of these historical precedents before considering what policies might work for our time.

We are not the only country with such a drug crisis. European countries have their drug crises as well: what are they doing? The issue of regulation should be investigated, as that is exactly the choice of one European country—the Netherlands. What sort of legalization have they put in place and what are the results? Briefly put, we need to know what has worked and what has not, the successful solutions and the attempts that failed. Beyond the general organization of considering history in this country and then taking a comparative look at Europe, this chapter will examine the primary drugs of concern.

Law Enforcement and the Legalization Debate

Today, arguments against the law enforcement option have made little headway. In 1964, at the very beginning of the contemporary drug crisis, an editorial appeared in *The Wall Street Journal*, written in agreement with a recommendation by the President's Advisory Committee. The editorial suggested that the Bureau of Narcotics be disbanded, for the Bureau, in the opinion of the editorial page, "...has become a symbol of a single theory of dealing with drug addiction. This theory rests on the premise that addiction is a crime and, for all practical purposes, little more than that."[1]

The quote is taken from Alfred R. Lindesmith's classic, *The Addict and the Law*. Lindesmith very much agreed with the Journal writer. The editorial pointed out the police option had been the government's approach to drug usage for at least half a century, that Washington bureaucrats' jobs were dependent on it remaining the nation's drug policy, and that bureaucracies such as the Bureau of Narcotics were the single most critical obstacle of necessary reform.[2] None of this is to say *The Wall Street Journal* is of the same opinion today.

Perhaps the writer of that editorial could have predicted no such action would be taken; instead the Bureau of Drug Abuse Control was created in 1966, then both bureaus were consolidated in 1968 into the Bureau of Narcotics and Dangerous Drugs within the Justice Department. Then that bureau, along with other bureaus with a role in drug enforcement, were consolidated into the Drug Enforcement Agency in 1973 as part of the Nixon administration's "all out global war on the drug menace."

The "current" drug crisis, the hyper-rhetoric of policymakers, and the law enforcement option have been with us for a rather long time. The fact that the drug crisis is continually worsening argues against the law enforcement option but, as polls show, that option remains popular and prudent politicians continue to stress it despite the results.

Most experts, however, as pointed out by Ethan Nadelmann in an article that appeared in *Foreign Policy* in the spring of 1988, favor understanding addiction and the drug issue as a health issue or, more generally, a social health issue, rather than as a criminal issue.[3] A typical example of the health approach can be found in the proceedings of the National Drug Abuse Conference of 1977.[4]

Here, one conferee argued that social class was a critical factor in drug abuse and that treatment programs should reflect this fact. Edward Kaufman argued that middle- and upper-class treatment should emphasize therapy and use the family as a resource, while treatment for underclass individuals must have a broader base, including providing for adequate housing, education, and jobs. In essence, his argument was that an effective treatment program must provide for underclass individuals what the family provides for the middle and upper-class individual. The lack of a family and community that can provide adequate housing, education, and job opportunities is, of course, what defines a person as underclass. This is a considerable extension of the health approach. The failure to take this social approach could well have sown the seeds for the current crisis.

This is not to say all expert commentators oppose current policy or that all who disagree with a given policy are in agreement with one another. For example, criminologist James Q. Wilson has written in favor of more expenditures for drug education and drug treatment while remaining in general agreement with the status quo. Criminologist James Inciardi has written in enthusiastic favor of current policy, only to back down somewhat in a recent work and call for more education and treatment.

Generally though, we have a case where expert opinion, favoring the health approach, and popular opinion, favoring the law enforcement approach, are quite opposite. One consequence of such a state of affairs is the timidity of public officials to even debate other possible options.

Former Secretary of State George Schultz in a recent public declaration favoring legalization of presently illicit drugs, or at least a debate on the issue, noted that he dared not say so while in office.

He stated: "Now that I am out of government I can say this," speaking to a group of alumni of the Stanford Business School. "We need at least to consider and examine forms of controlled legalization of drugs." He went on to say "No politician wants to say what I just said, not for a minute."[5]

However, there is one politician who while in office was willing to brave the tide of public opinion and Washington rhetoric and publicly raise the issue of legalization: Mayor Kurt Schmoke of Baltimore, at the U.S. Conference of Mayors in 1987.[6] Mayor Schmoke, a former federal prosecutor, did not call for legalization but rather for a debate on the merits of legalization in one form or another. As a result of his candor he was the only mayor of the nation's largest cities not asked to contribute to the present administration's report to Congress on drug strategies. But the other consequence was that legalization began to get some attention in the news media, a media that had otherwise, for the most part, solidly endorsed the administration's hysteria policy.[7]

Congress holds a position similar to the administration. Representative Charles Rangel (D-NY), chair of the Select Committee on Narcotics Abuse and Control, has closed the door to any such debate, stating: "I strongly object to even the mention of legalization as an option."[8] Still, according to one source, there is some silent support in Congress for a consideration of the issue.[9]

In academic circles, the leading advocate of the position that legalization should at least be debated is Ethan Nadelmann of Princeton University's Woodrow Wilson School of Public and International Affairs. He makes the argument that much of the evil associated with the current hysteria stems from the effects of the underground market rather than from the effects of drugs. He further argues that, for example, marijuana illegalization makes little sense when far more dangerous drugs such as alcohol and tobacco are legal.

Moreover, there have been others who have been actively advocating legalization. The major voices include economist and Nobel laureate Milton Friedman (who has advocated it since 1973); Lewis Lapham, editor of Harpers; William T. Burke, police chief of Portsmouth, New Hampshire; Federal Judge Robert W. Sweet; and Patrick Murphy, former police commissioner of New York City.

Their reasons for favoring legalization vary. Milton Friedman and William Buckley favor legalization on the grounds of individual liberty. Buckley adds that legalization will "...inevitably prevail because the alternatives are becoming increasingly discredited."[11]

However, this is not to say that the libertarians thereby favor the health approach.

The late psychiatrist and noted author Thomas Szasz offered the traditional libertarian argument in his 1974 work, *Ceremonial Chemistry*: "Autonomy is the death knell of authority and authority knows it...."[11] Hence, governmental authority is loath to regard the addict (or anyone) as a person capable of making a free choice. In Szasz's view, neither the liberal drug treatment clinic nor the jail is a satisfactory solution—for such policy options presume authority knows best and is rightfully empowered to overturn or rectify individual choice. Presumably, Milton Freidman and William Buckley would be sympathetic to this point of view.

Judge Sweet, holding another view and in a departure from the tradition of judicial silence on public issues, has stated that: "What we ought to do is try to get at the source of the problem, which is poverty and disillusion, and turn it around."[12]

The prime argument against regulating presently illicit drugs are concerns over the increase in addiction that might plausibly follow such legislation. In other words, in investigating the question of legalization, the question becomes: what would be the effects of enhanced availability?

We already know the opiate addiction rate prior to the illegalization of opiates, 3 percent, according to one rough estimate (3 percent is half our present day alcoholism rate).[13] However, we need a survey of what happens after a drug becomes decriminalized when it has never, for the generation in question, been legal. There is a history in this country of the decriminalization, if not outright legalization, of marijuana in eleven states—what does this history show?

A 1981 study by Dr. Deborah Maloff addressed this question. The study focused on reviewing the evidence from three states: California, Oregon, and Maine. The conclusions were that decriminalization had little effect on usage rates.[14] Indeed, from another study, there is some evidence that usage rates were lower in these states than in states that had not decriminalized.[15] Nonetheless, Dr. Maloff notes that "...existing research is lacking in both thoroughness and precision."[16]

Of course, there is the example of alcohol prohibition from 1919 to 1933. Here studies show a decrease of consumption during Prohibition and an increase following repeal. This is the general finding of such research. Though there are some contradictory claims, it is one of the more replicated findings of drug research that increased availability leads to increased usage and decreased availability leads to decreased usage. How can this be correlated with the just-noted decriminalization study?

The wide availability of marijuana (and cocaine, as well as other drugs) to high school and younger students was pointed out in an earlier chapter. Presumably, availability of drugs to youngsters is not appreciably different from availability to adults. Given such wide availability, decriminalization of marijuana probably may not increase availability to any appreciable degree. Hence, the general rule in this case is not invalid so much as irrelevant.

What of the second exception to the general rule, the Dutch example? Dutch youngsters, growing up in a country in which marijuana has long been decriminalized, show usage rates that are one-tenth American usage rates (by "usage rates" it is meant percentage of population reporting use).[17] The effect of making this drug as available as legal drugs has been to minimize the social appetite for the drug. This is not to claim that American marijuana use would decline to Dutch levels (or decline at all) following decriminalization.

The genie is out of the bottle, so to speak; the marijuana plant has acquired a mystique and a mythology that is not likely to be easily shed. Moreover, societies differ in their totality, not just in one particular way, so comparisons must always be tentative. We need only recall David Musto's thesis of America's particular liking for drugs (hence, the title of his work *The American Disease*) and that Americans consume 60 percent of the world's production of illicit drugs to appreciate that declines in usage are unlikely were a national policy of decriminalization to be instituted.

However, a complicating point is that increased availability may lead to increased usage as a general rule but the existence of laws that, paradoxically, increase demand may make for critical exceptions to the general rule. There is no absolutely stable and steady ground here for the law itself directly affects usage as well as availability. Nonetheless, the Dutch case has received much attention and will be further reviewed later.

Two Prohibitions: Alcohol and Cocaine

The next question regarding the supply-push of availability becomes: what of cocaine? Using alcohol (another addictive drug) as an example, we can expect cocaine usage to increase following regulation (even if regulation means only decriminalization of small amounts). But using the Dutch experience as a example, the Dutch people, according to one report, hardly use the drug despite the overall liberalism of their society.

If an answer is to be found, sensibly it should be found in a comparison between the previous and present history of cocaine usage in this country. For the purposes of further comparison, the history of alcohol prohibition will also be brought in.

Cocaine was once very popular in this country but then relatively disappeared for more than 70 years. The first cocaine fad was during the late nineteenth century. The use of cocaine in the original Coca-Cola is a widely known fact. Less well-known is the 1860s coca wine, "Vin Mariani," a wine endorsed by such people as President William McKinley and inventor Thomas Edison.[18] Cocaine itself was widely promoted by any number of individuals, including Sigmund Freud, who wrote a piece praising it to the hilt only to later retract his praise as its addictive potential and the problem of overdosage became more obvious.[19]

Reflecting the social psychology that is bound up in all drug use, cocaine was the drug of privilege and its use defined membership in the social elite. The image of cocaine was to change in the early twentieth century. The image of the "dope fiend" who was a danger to self and others was created at this time. Newspapers headlined the cocaine crazed African American male who committed crimes to get the drug and who committed yet more heinous crimes after partaking of the drug.

In short, the picture of cocaine was very much like that promoted today: after a time of being the signal drug of the privileged (during the 1970s), cocaine is now blamed for the latest crime wave, with crimes by African American males gaining special attention. One more parallel, the response to fears of the African American male and cocaine were the same, new and tougher drug laws. Regarding the earlier "drug crisis," the Harrison Drug Act was passed in 1914, outlawing opiates and cocaine.

Of further interest is that this Act worked. Cocaine use (along with opiate use), though never completely absent, was effectively curtailed by the Harrison Act and by the image promulgated by the media. This was the original Prohibition, law enforcement-based, and it worked.

There is some debate among researchers about what the Act meant. Lindesmith, in *The Addict and the Law*, argues that Congress did not mean to outlaw the drug so much as to ensure that only physicians could dispense the drug. Lindesmith argues that it was the Supreme Court, in the *U.S. v. Jin Fuey Moy* case, who interpreted the Act as a prohibition and, hence, made it one. Lindesmith argues that this was the first step down the road toward a rigid law enforcement approach and away from a flexible medical-based policy.[20]

Arnold S. Trebach, in *The Heroin Solution* (1982),[21] disputes this view, claiming Congress meant to impose a prohibition whatever the vagaries of the wording of the bill. Lindesmith points to the wording of the bill, Trebach to the Congressional Record and papers of the day. In either case, reformers then moved on to the next most dangerous drug—alcohol—and this drug was banned in 1919. This is the critical fact of alcohol: it is not widely available today because it is safe; it is widely available because Prohibition failed.

One prohibition worked and the other didn't—why? The relative success and failure of the two prohibitions (cocaine and opiates on one hand, alcohol on the other) cannot be found in the law or the law enforcement approach for in both cases the law and the police option were the same. The explanation of the success of one and the failure of the other is social.

Alcohol was acceptable to white mainstream culture; it was their drug of choice; cocaine was not. The media association of cocaine with African American males (rather than the affluent) and then the media association of African American males with crime and even fears of a revolution against southern whites, further diminished its attractiveness to white users in the era of Jim Crow.

Regarding opiates, these became associated with Asian-Americans at a time when this minority was the object of considerable and open prejudice. Likewise, in the late 1930s, when marijuana was prohibited, it was associated with African-Americans and Mexican-Americans, equally stigmatized populations. Such associations diminished the substance's social appeal, a factor as critical as any physiological effect in the patterns of drug use.

Additionally, and this was true of all drugs labeled "narcotics" by law but not by pharmacological effect, the people, press and politicians of the particular eras gave themselves the satisfaction of taking a hard and firm stand against drug use, and, biting the bullet, outlawed the other group's drug of choice. The same is exactly true today.

The current history of cocaine repeats the previous history. Originally a drug of the "elite," it became associated with African

American males. Fears of crime and fears of the African American male combined and the consequence was new and tougher drug laws. Further, following their passage, usage declined. Can it be concluded that usage will further decline and that cocaine usage will again become marginal?

This, in my opinion, is unlikely. As noted earlier, numbers of people reporting any usage is down, emergency room visits for "crack" overdoses are down, but numbers of people reporting weekly usage has increased and the estimates of total volume of cocaine imports are continually increasing.

Such contradictions can be reconciled if the increase in weekly users can account for reports of increased shipments. After all, 5 to 10 percent of alcohol users account for 50 percent of all alcohol sales.[22] Presumably, such a fact would be true for all drugs. On the other hand, a simpler explanation is that individuals are under-reporting their illegal usage, given the current atmosphere of hysteria against "drug users."

Cocaine imports may well decline as middle-class usage declines given the association of cocaine with the African American male. However, cocaine will not retreat to marginal levels. Usage will be bifurcated, with the underclass and upper-income groups providing the bulk of users. Underclass use will remain, for underclass neighborhoods have so few defenses against the supply-side. Upper-income use will continue as law enforcement efforts are weak against this group and further, this is the group that can well afford the drug.

David Musto, Yale historian and psychiatrist, wrote the standard text on drug legislation, *The American Disease*. This work has been frequently referred to here. Musto has a different argument to make regarding the future of the current "drug crisis." To Musto, there is a recurring pattern of drug usage. A particular drug is "discovered" and enthusiastic promotion of its virtues leads to increasing numbers of people experimenting with the drug. This leads to an era of tolerance that concludes when the long-term and negative effects of the drug become known. The reversal of public attitudes toward the drug brings the crisis to conclusion as increasing numbers of individuals stop (or never start) using the drug. Such a pattern describes the history of opiates, cocaine, marijuana, LSD, as well as other drugs. Musto concludes that the current hysteria will follow the same pattern.

The difficulty, in my opinion, is that there are exceptions to this general pattern. Sources of public information and education

about drugs include alcohol commercials, especially sports programming that encourages young people to indulge in alcohol.
Such programming is bound to undermine any anti-drug campaign
or, at best, transfer the social problem from one drug to another.
Contrary to Musto's general thesis, the alcohol problem has not
disappeared, it has been ignored by public authorities.

Further, as one commentator has maintained, among young people it is peers rather than the government that is the source of
information about drugs.[23] Young people look to one another for
information, rather than to public authorities. Moreover, a critical
and new feature of our time is that the underground market
includes the very young. Reaching this pre-adolescent market is
going to require special programs and a special effort—but the current administration considers drug education something of a waste
of time (William Bennett's position).

Moreover, many occasional (and frequent) users of drugs such as
marijuana and cocaine have been using them all of their adult
lives. If so, this is a distinct difference from earlier "fads" and one
that argues against the self-correcting mechanism found in Musto's
thesis.

On the other hand, the "crack" variant of cocaine will probably
follow Musto's predicted pattern. Both the evident danger of the
drug combined with its association with the underclass will serve
to bring the career of this drug to a close. Moreover, there is
already the example of "PCP," a once-popular drug that has nearly
disappeared as its dangers became recognized (and another drug
that followed Musto's pattern).

By no means will the crisis be over, however, as another drug
will be found to take its place. Indeed, this is already happening
with the appearance of a crystal form of methamphetamine, or
"ice". "Ice" is the African American underclass version of the
rural and white underclass stimulant and euphoric drug of choice,
"crank," also a form of methamphetamine.[24] The appeal of such
drugs is their cheapness and their opiate-like euphoric effect, an
effect achieved without needle injection.

The Comparative Case: The Dutch

The Dutch have followed a policy of decriminalization since
1976. Though it is not legal to sell or possess marijuana, the laws
against it are not enforced: "You can smoke a joint on the steps of
police headquarters and never be arrested," a Dutch Justice

Ministry official is quoted as saying in a *Los Angeles Times* article.[25]

Marijuana is openly sold without police reaction. Most "soft" drugs such as marijuana and hashish are sold in "coffee shops." Amsterdam itself has more than 350 such shops. This may seem to be a large number and an easy temptation for youth. The facts are quite the reverse. In a 1984 survey of Dutch high school students, only 6 percent stated they had used marijuana in the previous year. This is one-tenth the U.S. rate for that year.[26] Evidently, illegalization adds a certain mystique to marijuana and hashish for U.S. youth, a mystique utterly lacking for Dutch youth.

Openness is also the policy regarding "hard" drugs such as cocaine and heroin. The Dutch again do not take a law enforcement approach toward small amounts, encouraging their addicts to "surface" and providing methadone on demand as well as needles from mobile treatment vans. One result is that the ugliness of the fact of addiction is highly visible: junkies openly shoot up on the street and prostitution is rampant.

Nonetheless, no arrests are made unless non-addicts are harassed or adulterated drugs are being sold. Further, American cities are not spared such ugliness, even with a hard-line approach. The Dutch consider the degraded appearance of the addict to itself be a deterrent to would-be youthful users.[27]

At one time, hard drugs could be openly sold. This practice was stopped (things got rapidly out of hand), but the open selling of soft drugs continues to be permitted. The Dutch once provided methadone to all, including foreigners, but now foreigners are bused back to their country of origin. Further, there is treatment on demand for all Dutch citizens.

What are the consequences of such a policy? First of all, only the Netherlands and Singapore can report a drop in the number of addicts (the policy of the Singapore government could not be more different: they have the death penalty for sellers of hard drugs). The average age of addicts is getting higher (from 26 to 31), indicating a decline in overall numbers as fewer young people are reported to be addicts.

Moreover, the Netherlands is one of the few places thought to have a handle on their AIDS problem. The policy of encouraging users to surface and providing on demand treatment appears to have stabilized the AIDS epidemic. Also, there has been no appearance of "crack," the plague of the American underclass. Another benefit is that accurate epidemiological data can be collected.

Addicts are required to register with public health authorities to gain free treatment. Therefore, the Dutch know just how much of a problem they have.

This is quite unlike the situation in our own country, where there is an utter lack of reliable data on the extent of the hard drug problem. Of course, there is a downside to permitting addicts to surface. One Dutch official noted: "This worsens our cosmetic problem. The paradox now is that it looks worse now than before."[28] However, even this may have benefits: "They are a very visible lesson for those who see them, a living anti-drug argument."[29]

Dutch drug policy director Eddy Engelsman states that the Dutch policy is supported by both liberals and conservatives.[30] Nonetheless, dissenting opinions can be found. In 1984, Police Deputy Chief Evert Jagerman of Amsterdam was quoted as saying: "We have been too tolerant. We don't arrest users of heroin because there isn't enough capacity in the jails. People who steal get sent back on the street again. We arrest the same people over and over."[31]

In addition, some 90 percent of Amsterdam's street crime has been attributed to heroin addicts. Still, Dutch crime statistics remain at European levels, and in no way approach American crime rates. Nonetheless, heroin addicts apparently produce the same sort of problems whether a liberal health approach or conservative law and order approach is used. Still, the health approach of the Dutch is reducing the numbers of addicts as well as providing a reliable measure of the problem.

Both the law enforcement and the health approach are found in public policy. Hard drugs are actively kept out of the country with a rigorous law enforcement policy. Large-scale dealers are busted yet users are tolerated, in that they are treated as unfortunate people with a severe health problem rather than as criminals.

A report released by the U.S. Embassy in The Hague noted: "Finally and when possible, it assists his eventual reintegration into society. The policy is often mistranslated and misinterpreted as 'indulgent' or 'permissive.' In fact, in this society, it acts as a powerful social control."[32] The report was dismissed by American officials in Washington.

The core of the Dutch policy is to set priorities, with the prime priority being the separation of hard drugs from soft drugs. The American report noted that the aim of the Dutch policy is to reduce the harm the addicted population can bring to the rest of the population (via crimes of theft, for example). Amsterdam Mayor Eduard van Thijn states: "We have a pragmatic policy. On the one hand, we reject legalization of hard drugs very strongly, because that is surrender. But we also reject a policy of total war, which is overkill."[33]

He goes on to add: "The secret to our pragmatic policy is this distinction between hard and soft drugs. In Amsterdam, the two scenes have been completely separated. We have proven that the stepping-stone theory doesn't work, that soft drugs do not necessarily lead to hard drugs."[34] This is consistent with recent research in this country on the effects of casual usage.

The Dutch label their drug policy "normalization." By this, the director of Dutch policy explains: "It is a normal problem...one of various problems a society is faced with."[35] He goes on to add that a "normalization" approach opposes "...putting it [the drug problem] on a pedestal and saying our society is at stake."[36] Hence, the policy is deliberately anti-hysterical and stresses flexibility and pragmatism. This means treating the problem as a health problem rather than strictly a law enforcement problem.

A report by Malcolm Dean, appearing in the British medical journal *The Lancet*, a source used above, compared the outcome of Dutch and German drug policies. The German policy is hard-line, similar to the American policy. The outcome: the Germans' have an increasing crime rate, three times the per capita number of addicts and twice the number of over-doses as the Dutch. Dean writes: "Thirteen years ago, Dutch policy-makers set themselves three goals: the separation of soft and hard drugs; the deglamorizing of hard-drug addiction; and the integration of drug programmes with other addiction schemes for alcoholics and smokers...All three goals have been achieved."[37]

The key question becomes, can such an experience be duplicated in America? It is quite implausible that the usage by American youth of marijuana would drop to 6 percent following decriminalization. Nonetheless, decriminalization would diminish that mystique, or at least stop propagating it, and would represent the establishment of priorities, the lack of which is a striking failure of American policy.

Regarding heroin and the policy of treatment on demand, mobile methadone clinics, and clean needles, the health rather than law enforcement approach has produced a remarkable success story for the Dutch (relative to other countries' success with managing their addicted population and minimizing the harm such populations can cause others). Moreover, by having a list of registered addicts, the Dutch public health system has a hard and accurate count on the number of addicts. Unlike us, they know for sure the dimensions of the problem. Of course, given the lack of a national public health system, Americans neither know the number of drug treatment clinics in the country, nor the numbers receiving treatment. Lack of basic information provides further fuel for hysteria. One possible approach is to borrow this much of Dutch policy (treatment on demand and needle exchange), while rejecting the open acceptance of addiction.

Is there any evidence from an American setting that we can use instead of plausible predictions? There is one example: the distribution of clean needles has been tried in New York City. Unfortunately, by most accounts, few addicts were interested.[38] Critics note that the needles were distributed outside jails and police stations, not exactly the most promising places if one truly wanted access to this population. Not only would a greater effort be required to reach this population but a more thoroughgoing reorientation toward a health approach would have to take place. Nonetheless, from this one experiment and these reports, it appears a weak health approach combined with an aggressive law-enforcement approach toward the same population is bound to fail.

However, there is a strong dissenting opinion regarding the New York experiment, an opinion that the experiment worked well enough to be worth further trial. One proponent maintains that there was an imposed quota of 200 addicts, hence the low number of enrollees given by the media is a politically created fact. Also, the claim is made that 78 percent of the addicts accepted referral to a drug treatment clinic. Of further interest, 51 percent of the enrollees tested positive for the HIV antibody.[39]

Again, such reaching out would not be for the sake of the addict per se. The hard-core addict has evidently lost all sense of individual judgement and sensibility and without this innate healer no successful treatment of the individual use problem is possible. The point of reaching out is to minimize the harm to others that addicts can cause.

One further point: the policy of giving away clean needles is equally unpopular with the general public and with politicians. The dispensing of clean needles has been recommended by experts to diminish the rate of AIDS found in the addicted population and the spread of this disease to the non-addicted populations via the use of addicted prostitutes.[40]

This can be understood as part of a general reluctance to really face up to this crisis; however hot the rhetoric, little funding follows save for the police. Methadone maintenance is available to only a few of those who seek and might benefit from the treatment. Likewise, drug treatment facilities, as previously noted, are meager in this country for those who cannot afford private treatment. These deficiencies can be trusted to continue to maintain the heroin problem, however much money is thrown at it via law enforcement.

None of this is to say that the health approach, minimally put as medicalizing the problem, will eliminate the problem of heroin addiction or the crime associated with that addiction. The Dutch have made a successful effort to diminish the problem but at the cost of turning Amsterdam into an eyesore, at least in the opinion of many. Of course, it is unclear if American cities are any prettier. The conservative approach here may well be producing the same sort of problem as the very liberal approach of the Dutch. Returning to the main point, the Dutch harbor no illusions about curing the problem of addiction and rightfully so; no treatment approach has ever shown more than limited success.

What of the English approach to the heroin problem? Edwin Schur, in a classic comparative work published in 1962 (*Narcotics in Britain and the U.S.*), highly praised the English system of heroin maintenance (the dispensing of heroin to registered addicts). However, a rise in addiction rates led the British to suspend that practice and substitute heroin maintenance. Such a change was not the outcome of legislated law; instead health professionals initiated and executed the policy change by a consensus among themselves. Despite the change, the rise in addiction apparently continued, combined with a resurgence in the underground market.[41]

Arnold Trebach has pointed out the difficulties in drawing conclusions from the British practice. First, the doctor-patient relationship in England is a more privileged relationship than is permitted in the United States. There are far fewer legal constraints regarding the doctor's advice and treatment. Whatever the merits of such privilege, this means policy execution is unclear, given the greater authority of individual physicians to act on their own. Therefore, it is difficult to know just what a particular policy, such as the policy on heroin treatment, really is.

Furthermore, English policy as defined by the Health Ministry has changed over the years and has never been uncontroversial.

Despite enthusiastic reports here of English success in regard to their heroin problem, the English themselves are considerably more skeptical about any such "success." From a report more recent than Trebach's, the one thing English professionals appear to agree on is that the American "war against drugs" is nonsensical and doomed to fail.[42]

At this date, the English prefer a pragmatic policy quite similar to the Dutch. Heroin or methadone maintenance is still available but the preferred treatment is detoxification. The English seek "harm reduction," reducing the potential harm of the addiction to the user by offering needle exchanges and education in how to respond to overdoses. Given that the addict is more underground in England than in Amsterdam (given that maintenance programs have, for the most part, given way to detoxification treatment, the user goes to the underground market for supplies), the statistics that would measure success are obscure. Nonetheless, English crime statistics remain at European rather than American levels and the problem of AIDS is far greater here.

Heroin (or morphine) would appear to be the exception to the general argument presented here. The sociological and the social-psychological apparently take a back seat to the pharmacological, with the euphoria produced by heroin overwhelming social considerations. Picking up this question leads to perhaps the oldest debate in drug policy literature: the role of the Harrison Act in generating the current problem.

Essentially, the argument (most forcefully put by Lindesmith) runs as follows: before the Harrison Act, the addicted person was as often found in upper social circles as in lower and pitied as a person with a terrible health problem, rather than condemned as morally derelict. After the Harrison Act, heroin addiction was eventually confined nearly exclusively to the lower-income class and, in addition, the addiction was considered a moral stigma.

This change was due to a series of facts stemming from the Act. First, the upper-income groups eventually stopped using after the Act was passed and after the image of the degraded lower-income user became indelibly pressed into the public mind as part of that era's "war against drugs." The upper classes stopped using but members of the lower class were undeterred by either prison or stigmatization. In this way, the current problem was created. The illegalization of heroin/morphine supplies completed the evolution of the user as the addicted became tied to the underground market for supplies and to criminality itself for income.

The counterargument, perhaps most forcefully put by James Inciardi, is simply that the pharmacological effects of the drug create the degraded user. In my opinion, this is a case where each argument has merit on its own terms. The sociological argument of Lindesmith and others explains the broad history of heroin addiction, the shift in the sort of user, as well as the shift in the general understanding and picture of the user. The counterargument addresses directly the narrower issue of the problem of heroin addiction.

There is no stable point of reference in determining the relative safety and dangers of drugs, particularly when cultural understandings are mixed into the equation. For example, remember the opening point in regard to alcohol and how different cultural understandings about alcohol by the Jewish person and the non-Jewish person greatly diminishes the danger of alcohol to the Jewish person. Nonetheless, the fact of injection and the danger of it greatly increases the risk factor of heroin, whatever the sociological facts. Further, when the risk of AIDS, a new risk, is added to the equation, the relevance of the old debate appears to diminish. The need is to directly confront the problem. Regretfully, the paralysis of Washington policymakers remains unchanged.

Drug Laws and Social Facts

The general interpretation of Prohibition, such as can be found in Samuel Eliot Morrison's *History of the American People*, is that alcohol prohibition represented not simply an issue about drug usage but rather represented the clash of cultural values and the striving of one cultural group to assert dominance over another.

In the case of Prohibition, the argument is that the upsurge in Catholic immigrants had become a threat to the continued dominance of Protestant culture in America. Alcohol use was just as much symbolic of that cultural clash as it was a substantive issue; alcohol usage being much more tolerated among Catholics than among Protestants. The real question was not alcohol use, but what culture was to be the governing culture of the country, Catholic or Protestant? Protestant America had the power to enact Prohibition but not the power to make it effective.

Likewise, marijuana prohibition can be understood in the very same way. Here the clash of cultures is not ethnic but a clash across generations. The same culture, the so-called "counterculture," that favored the use of marijuana was also the culture that was challenging the status quo in any number of ways, marijuana being perhaps the most trivial of the challenges.

Marijuana, like alcohol to the earlier generation, was a substantive issue, but it was much more a symbolic issue of that larger clash between culture and counterculture. Furthermore, the question was the same: what culture and what values were to govern America? Likewise, the outcome was the same as the earlier alcohol prohibition. The culture in power had the power to maintain the prohibition but not the power to make it effective in any meaningful way.

"Drug" usage readily becomes symbolic of larger issues and these issues are more truly based in culture and cultural clashes than in any sort of balanced and reasoned assessment of risks and benefits. This explains why expert opinion is so little listened to in the current drug crisis and why the law enforcement option is being pursued to such an extreme degree, even as its failure and the many problems associated with it become ever more apparent. The issue is culture and what culture is to govern.

In this sense, the issue is equally one of power. This is why the law enforcement option is pursued even to the point of diminishing constitutional liberties and openly advocating the further reduction of individual liberty (such has been explicitly called for by William Bennett). When the issue is power itself, then the diminution of individual liberty can become tolerated (at least by those who favor the status quo), for it is governmental power itself that is felt to be in jeopardy. Further, given conflicting cultures, the implicit understanding is that the cutback in liberties will only happen to members of a particular subculture and not all members.

Evidence of this larger symbolic issue comes from analyses of Mr. Reagan and his pronouncements while in office. Mr. Reagan often seemed to want to re-fight the "sixties," or at least to pretend, more or less, that they never happened. Such an attitude, surely not unique to Mr. Reagan, is representative of the opinion of the larger culture and it is an opinion compatible with a cultural analysis of marijuana prohibition. To accept marijuana would be to accept the counterculture. The antagonisms and controversies of that era have not ended but rather have gone underground to emerge in symbolic forms.

We are a society of change. To one generation, alcohol and tobacco use is absolutely understandable and acceptable whatever the social and individual costs, but all other drugs are "narcotics" and bad. Yet to another generation, marijuana use is perfectly acceptable while alcohol use is questionable and even, in the case of tobacco, highly stigmatized. Yet, at the same time, both generations co-exist and the legal and criminal justice system is expected to straighten out the contradictions by the application of coercion.

Perhaps it is change itself that is feared. But such changes are to be expected in a world in which the social sphere undergoes transformations as dramatic and thorough as the technological sphere. Such thoroughgoing changes are sure to wreak havoc in any criminal justice system that attempts to reflect and mold that social sphere via dogmatic and coercive policies.

According to Amitri Etizoni, even as the potential has expanded for unintended consequences, so too has the potential for deliberate change. To enact positive change, pragmatic judgement and a persistent, thoroughgoing effort to get at the roots as well as the branches of the problem is called for. In other words, there must be an appreciation for the larger social milieu within which laws and law-enforcement operate, and this must replace the empty-minded rhetoric that characterizes the current policy and current failure.

Notes

1. Alfred Lindesmith, *The Addict and the Law* (Bloomington: Indiana University Press, 1965), 243.
2. Ibid.
3. Ethan A. Nadalmann, "U.S. Drug Policy: A Bad Export," *Foreign Policy* 70 (Spring 1988): 83-108.
4. David Smith, *A Multicultural View of Drug Abuse* (Cambridge: Schenkman, 1978).
5. "Drug Legalization: Interest Rises in Prestigious Circles," *Los Angeles Times*, 20 November 1989, A 18.
6. Ibid.
7. Ibid.
8. Eliot Marshall, "Legalization Gets a Hearing," *Science* 241 (September 1988): 1158.
9. Ibid.
10. "Legalizing Drugs: Failures Spur Debate," *New York Times*, 27 November 1989, A 9:4.
11. Thomas Szasz, *Ceremonial Chemistry: The Ritual Persecution of Drugs, Addicts and Pushers* (Garden City, NY: Anchor Press, 1974), 175.
12. "Taking on the Legalizers," Newsweek, 25 December 1989, 46.
13. This estimate is taken from Troy Duster, *The Legislation of Morality* (New York: The Free Press, 1970). Duster's estimate comes from a

compilation and comparison of a number of studies on the topic. Arnold Taylor also addressed the question in *American Diplomacy and the Narcotics Traffic 1900-1939*,125-26.

14. Deborah Maloff, "A Review of the Effects of the Decriminalization of Marijuana," *Contemporary Drug Problems* 10 (Fall 1981): 307-21.

15. L. Johnston, "Marijuana use and the effects of marijuana decriminalization," testimony delivered at hearings on the effects of marijuana, Senate Subcommittee on Criminal Justice, Judiciary Committee, 16 January 1980, 307-21. From Deborah Maloff, "A Review of the Effects of the Decriminalization of Marijuana," *Contemporary Drug Problems* 10 (Fall 1981): 307-21.

16. Deborah Maloff, "A Review of the Effects of the Decriminalization of Marijuana," *Contemporary Drug Problems* 10 (Fall 1981): 307-21.

17. Malcolm Dean, "The Dutch Soft-Drug Policy," *Lancet* 334 (21 October 1989): 993-94. The same figure was also given by the Dutch Director of the Alcohol, Drugs and Tobacco Branch of the Dutch Health Ministry, Eddy Engelsman, in a filmed interview with Arnold Trebach, President of the Drug Policy Foundation (Washington DC). This is found in the video Do the Dutch Do It Better? (Washington, DC: Drug Policy Foundation, 1990) in the series America's Drug Forum.

18. Ronald K. Siegel, "Cocaine and the Privileged Class," *Advances in Alcohol and Substance Abuse*, 4(2) (Winter 1984): 42.

19. Weldon Witters and Peter Venturelli, *Drugs and Society* (Boston: Jones and Bartlett, 1988, 152.

20. Alfred Lindesmith, *The Addict and the Law*, 3-35.

21. Arnold S. Trebach, *The Heroin Solution* (New Haven: Yale Press, 1982).

22. The 5 percent figure comes from Marcia Russell, Cynthia Henderson and Sheila B. Blume, *Children of Alcoholics: A Review of the Literature* (Buffalo: New York State Division of Alcoholism and Alcohol Abuse, Research Institute on Alcoholism, 1985). The 10 percent figure comes from NIAAA, Sixth Annual Report to the U.S. Congress on Alcohol and Health, DHHS Pub. No. 97-1519, (Washington, DC: U.S. Government Printing Office, 1985). I submit both figures here.

23. David Forbes, "Saying No to Ron and Nancy: School-Based Drug Abuse Prevention Programs in the 1980's," *Journal of Education* 169 (1987): 80-90.

24. It is unclear from the research if "crank" is the same form of methamphetamine as "ice" or a variant of the same drug.

25. "Drugs: Dutch Gain with Tolerant Tack," *Los Angeles Times*, 22 September 1989, 10.

26. Malcolm Dean, "The Dutch Soft-Drug Policy," *Lancet*, 334 (21 October 1989): 993-94. Malcolm Dean is the Guardian's social policy leader-writer. In addition, see note 17. For a recent report that includes the Malaysian experience (a hard-line approach that is failing), see "Intensive War on Drugs by Malaysia and Singapore Shows Mixed Results," New York Times, 15 December 1989. Scott B.

Macdonald, *Dancing on a Volcano: The Latin-American Drug Trade* (New York: Praeger, 1988) also includes a summary of reports from Europe and Asia.

27. Malcolm Dean, "The Dutch Soft-Drug Policy," *Lancet* 334 (21 October 1989): 993-94.
28. "Drugs: Dutch Gain with Tolerant Tack," *Los Angeles Times*, 22 September 1989, 11.
29. Ibid.
30. The Dutch Director of the Alcohol, Drugs and Tobacco Branch of the Dutch Health Ministry, Eddy Engelsman, in a filmed interview with Arnold Trebach, President of the Drug Policy Foundation (Washington DC). This is found in the video *Do the Dutch Do It Better?* (Washington DC: Drug Policy Foundation, 1990) in the series America's *Drug Forum.*"
31. Rosemary Brady, "In Dutch," Forbes, 27 February 1984, 46.
32. "Drugs: Dutch Gain with Tolerant Tack," *Los Angeles Times*, 22 September 1989, A11.
33. Ibid., A10.
34. Ibid.
35. The Dutch Director of the Alcohol, Drugs and Tobacco Branch of the Dutch Health Ministry, Eddy Engelsman, in a filmed interview with Arnold Trebach, President of the Drug Policy Foundation (Washington DC). This is found in the video Do the Dutch Do It Better? (Washington DC: Drug Policy Foundation, 1990) in the series America's Drug Forum."
36. Ibid.
37. Malcolm Dean, "The Dutch Soft-Drug Policy."
38. "Needle Plan Fails to Attract Drug Addicts So Its Revised," *New York Times*, 30 January 1989. Also see "Addicts to Get Needles in Plan to Curb AIDS," *New York Times*, 31 January 1988.
39. Gillman, Cherni, "New York City's Needle Exchange Experiment: Policy Implications From It's First Year" in *Research Monograph No. 105, NIDA, Problems of Drug Dependence 1990: Proceedings of the 52nd Annual Scientific Meeting of the Committee on Problems of Drug Dependence* (Washington, DC: Government Printing Office, 1990).
40. Timothy F. Kirn, 21 October 1988. "Drug Abuse: More Help Available for Addicted Persons But Main Problem Continues Unabated," *Journal of the American Medical Association* 260, no. 15 (21 October 1988): 2170-72.
41. John Jay Rouse and Bruce D. Johnson, "Hidden Paradigms of Morality in Debates About Drugs: Historical and Policy Shifts in British and American Drug Policy." In *The Drug Legalization Debate*, ed. James Inciardi. (Newbury Park, CA; Sage, 1991).
42. Rouse, "Hidden Paradigms of Morality in Debates About Drugs."

9

Summary, Nine Social Facts, and Policy Proposals

Is there a "drug crisis"? Given that Americans consume 60 percent of the world's production of all illicit drugs (and 80 percent of the world's production of cocaine), that the annual spending for legal and illegal mood/behavioral drugs in this country is approximately 170 billion dollars (a conservative estimate), the extraordinary measures proposed by the government to discourage such behavior (in its illicit forms), the consequences of such measures and the sheer volume of newsprint and television time spent encouraging the general hysteria (instead of, for example, presenting the facts)—this makes the "drug crisis" an enormous social fact, worthy of taking some time to understand, quite apart from any estimation of the genuineness or spuriousness of the "crisis" as conventionally defined.

The frame of this argument has been to identify those factors generating the crisis: the medicine society that generates the demand for the goods of the underground market, the internationalization of that demand, and the leisure and personality society that tolerates such preferences. A continuing theme is that society has changed, the infrastructure of values, beliefs, and practices has changed, yet the superstructure of law and policy has not. A parallel was drawn between the "stagflation" economic crisis of the 1970s and the social "drug crisis" of the 1980s, both examples of the consequences of meeting new challenges with traditional but outmoded responses.

In this view, commentators tell us we are moving away from the industrial society to some other sort of world, often characterized as post-modern. In this society that is still becoming, behavioral drug use will be tolerated, even by individuals who do not themselves use such drugs. Moreover, this new society is a society without a mainstream save in myth; individuals will look to their small and self-selected social groups for their values. In such a society, hard-line law regarding individual behavior is bound to be controversial and widely disregarded. In addition, the question might be asked, how is this so different from what has always been the case? It is a traditional American value to disregard inconvenient laws (as demonstrated in the indictments of Reagan administration officials as well as savings and loan executives).

Moreover, the combination of the generous consumption of behavioral drugs combined with laws that prohibit such consumption is evidence of collective denial. Drugs are not safe, but given laws such as the legalization of alcohol and tobacco, drugs that together account for a half million deaths annually, combined with the illegalization of far less lethal drugs—such contradictions in the law take a social toll. That toll is the drug crisis.

These are not the only sorts of contradictions that could be noted. It is perfectly legal to purchase an assault rifle and all of the ammunition one could want, but it is thought that a bowl of marijuana is far too dangerous to be permitted to be in anyone's hands. Given such contradictions, how can the public be surprised that drug laws are ignored?

Further, there are institutions at hand, public health institutions and law enforcement agencies that are the vehicles of social control, to contain the crisis. How are they doing? The public health system, if such a word is appropriate for the haphazard collection of public health agencies that only in a writer's imagination could be called a "system," is itself in crisis. Rather than a tool for containing the drug crisis, its own inadequacies, including but not limited to the absence of drug treatment programs and public health information, help fuel the crisis.

The law enforcement approach is a failure. Moreover, expert advice need not be taken at face value. The policy has been tried in Washington, D.C. and it failed. The effects of police action, particularly "effective" police action, is to continually displace the problem into other locations and onto other drugs without ever getting at the roots of the problem.

Moreover, the hypocrisy of policy, the ignoring of the role of the influential (including government agencies) in generating the crisis while focusing law enforcement on the most vulnerable members of the society—the underclass—has only exacerbated far older wounds than the drug crisis.

Meanwhile, the existence of an underground market has become a greater problem than the problem drug laws were meant to address. The government of the Soviet Union, with unlimited police authority (before *perestroika*), was unable to contain its underground market. Therefore, one must wonder how we can believe we can control our own solely by law enforcement measures?

Furthermore, the expansion of the authority of police agencies and the Federal government over everyday life has led to the overwhelming of the courts, the filling of the prisons and the whittling down of individual liberty and constitutional protections. The United States now imprisons more of its people per capita than any other nation in the world. Yet current policy calls for imprisoning yet more Americans. This policy is being actively carried out by the courts—witness the dramatic increases in the numbers of Americans arrested and placed behind bars—yet the crisis continues without significant change.

There remains the more fundamental problem, that once a government gains enhanced power over the lives of citizens, police, and governmental authorities are loath to cut such authority back.

What has prevented the crisis from spreading further? The natural healer, without which no remedy is possible, is individual judgement and decision-making. The vast majority of individuals restrain their usage. Further, in many cases, individual sensibility is expressed by seeking help for the problem of drug use that individuals are unable to deal with on their own. But there is a class for which no such treatment is available: the underclass.

Given this, we would expect the worst of the crisis to be found in the underclass and we do. It is proposed that the traditional resources, drug education and drug treatment, be given greater emphasis than the law enforcement option. Any drug regulation of whatever sort will require law enforcement, but law enforcement should be the last resort instead of being the first and only resort.

Moreover, it was also recommended that businesses hire high school athletes, individuals who are highly sought by underclass drug marketeers. Another recommendation was that police authorities should look to the "urban villagers" as potentially valuable allies in police efforts to contain violent gangs. Last, in our rush to apply draconian, highly technological and expensive measures, we have overlooked the simple, human solution—like the dedication of individuals such as Officer Kilroy. Such individuals should be sought out and encouraged.

However important drug treatment and education programs are, as well as business and police outreach programs (and they are, in my opinion, quite important), they will not be enough. There is an issue of social justice here. To be without health care is to be outside the American system. The pride of American society is its medicine. Those without access to that medicine are effectively cut off from the benefits of the American system while being vulnerable to its worst side—the application of police power to what are essentially social, rather than criminal, problems.

Pursuing this latter point: in this way, the police station becomes the emergency room of America's social ills. But the stationhouse cannot remedy those social ills. Perhaps it is thought that only the poor are shortchanged. The fact is every American is made poorer: the American who fears to walk the streets at night, the American who fears for the health and safety of his or her children at school, and the American who pays the bills for the lack of a genuine safety net.

This argument can be explicitly put in terms of nine social facts which will lead to policy recommendations. They are as follows:

(1) *The first fact is the ambiguity of the crisis.*

Any estimation of social "crisis" is normative rather than objective. Even when consensus can be reached that a crisis exists, agreement on the nature of the crisis can be hard to find. In the case of the drug crisis, government officials maintain there is a crisis of usage. However, critics such as Arnold Trebach and Ethan Nadelmann maintain the real crisis is created by the laws and the underground market the laws have created and maintained.

Regarding usage levels, such levels have retreated to the levels of 1973, the same year Richard Nixon called for "an all out global war against the drug menace." That speech was greeted with yawns. Today, nearly the same usage levels have the words "menace," "epidemic," and "scourge" on everyone's lips. In addition, 3 percent of the population reports weekly use of cocaine and this is taken as concrete evidence of an "epidemic." Yet if the same standard were applied to alcohol, a drug with all if not more of the harmful physical and psychological effects of cocaine, some 60 percent to 70 percent of the population would thereby be classified as "alcoholics."

The government's role is made yet more ambiguous given persistent and in many cases undenied stories of Federal complicity in the drug trade. The "war" is an ambiguous one. On one hand, the Reagan administration publicly proclaimed a "war against drugs." On the other hand, in secrecy, administration officials were actively collaborating with international drug marketeers.

Nonetheless, the many public proclamations of a "war" has led to a war mentality, itself producing ambiguous results. The war mentality is followed to a logical conclusion by local police. For example, 50 pounds of cocaine was sold in a Cleveland neighborhood by a police collaborator in order to stop the sale of cocaine in the neighborhood.[1]. The police chief there still maintains there was no contradiction in the action. The same is true in international actions. For example, in order to curb drug shipments, a Colombian drug chieftain was hunted down even though the consequence of the effort was an increase in the supply of cocaine reaching the states.

(2) *Who defines the drug crisis? It is middle and uppermiddle class individuals who define the crisis and bring to their definition the particular biases of their class. The unintended consequences of this bias is to worsen the crisis.*

This means, for example, that prescription drug abuse, abuse that is responsible for more deaths than all illicit drugs combined, is mentioned nowhere as part of the drug crisis. This is solely because there are hardly any middle and uppermiddle class homes without drugs such as sedative/hypnotics in the family medicine cabinet. It is unthinkable to such individuals, any number of whom are public officials, that their drug of choice has anything to do with the drug crisis. Given that this is the class that generates the drug laws, their own drug preferences have been carefully excluded from scrutiny and illegalization. In other words, the bias directs what shall be considered part of the "drug crisis" and what shall not.

Such bias is further evidenced in drug-testing, where the rationale is offered that individuals must be tested for drugs when the performance of their job is related to the public safety. This strikes me as quite reasonable. However, what is remarkable is that none of this drug testing includes alcohol.

A worker such as an airline pilot, a railroad engineer or a bus driver, a police officer or fire fighter, all could be legally intoxicated on duty yet are not tested for this drug; only illicit drugs are tested for. How can this make sense? It only makes sense when one considers the biases and personal drug usage of the individuals defining the crisis.

A marvelous example of this comes from a story appearing in the *New York Times* in March 1990. A Federal Aviation Agency inspector talked with a cockpit crew for over an hour and then allowed the crew to fly a Boeing 727 with 91 passengers aboard, despite receiving a tip that the crew had been drinking prior to the flight. The crew flew from Fargo, N.D., to Minneapolis where they were arrested by another FAA inspector for being intoxicated and violating safety regulations. No doubt, were an illegal drug involved, the first inspector would never have let the plane leave the ground.[2]

Moreover, note again this fact of the medicine society: all the rationalizations and encouragements to use legal behavioral drugs easily translate into the same rationalizations and encouragements to use drugs defined as illegal. The alcohol industry spends billions of dollars each year convincing young people that alcohol use equals being social, that using alcohol means having friends and enjoying oneself. Such subtle but pervasive encouragements also translate into encouragements for individuals to use illicit drugs for the same purpose.

Further, as mentioned above, such promotions are for a drug, alcohol, that cannot be legally purchased by individuals under 21 (of course, the specific prohibition varies given different and changing regulations), hence, socialization into drinking alcohol becomes socialization into breaking the law regarding drug usage. Reducing such promotions would not cost the public treasury a single penny, yet not a political leader or administrator can be found who has proposed to do such a thing. The reasons for this are no mystery: alcohol and tobacco are the drugs of choice of the individuals who serve as politicians and bureaucrats.

However, it would be naive to overlook the contributions of the alcohol and tobacco industries to political campaigns as a factor in the blind eye public officials turn to the harm these drugs do. For example, in California, the tobacco industry is the largest single contributor to political campaigns. The industry contributes 100 times more money to political candidates today than 15 years ago.[3]

Current law and policy is not the outcome of a rational weighing of risks and benefits, unless one means the political costs of standing up to hysteria and the benefits of advocating the status quo. Similarly, the media's refusal to take a critical look at alcohol, combined with their partnership in promoting the general hysteria against all other drugs, is consistent with the importance of alcohol and tobacco ads to their revenues.

(3) *Expert advice is available regarding the "drug crisis." This advice, from academics, social commentators, medical professionals and police chiefs, is surprisingly unanimous yet is entirely ignored by both public officials and the public in general. The opinion of these experts is that current policy is a failure and that to achieve success the underlying conditions producing the crisis must be treated. Beyond the medicine society, America has a terrible underclass problem and the drug crisis is but one manifestation of that problem.*

Much has been made by administration officials of a recent increase in the price of cocaine as evidence of the success of the "war." It is pointed out that the price of cocaine in 1990 was $15,000 a kilo, while in 1989 the price was $10,000 to $12,000 a kilo. The increase is attributed to the success of law enforcement.[4]

What is entirely overlooked however is that as recently as 1986 the street price of cocaine was $35,000 (and in 1981, $60,000).[5] Such statistics, when looked at in their totality, are hardly evidence of success. Moreover, even as there have been real declines in usage rates, such rates remain near historical highs and there is no evidence that law enforcement is responsible for the declines. Further, new sorts of problems are appearing, such as the increasing use of alcohol by young children.

The argument presented in this work is consistent with expert advice, advice that states attention should be given to the underclass and the demand generated by "the medicine society." Such advice is ignored exactly because such a course of action would conflict with political expediency. When in conflict with other priorities, social and public health comes in a distant second. Consequently, we have little of either.

The medicine society has been extensively detailed. This section focuses on the underclass. Some 20 percent of the American population lives in third world conditions. There is a concentration of social problems in this class; increasing problematic drug usage is only one of a range of problems. Refusing to address these problems is creating, as any number of experts have noted, a "lost generation" of individuals who have little chance of becoming middle-class and, probably, little desire to do so. Like the budget deficit, such social problems are simply being passed on to the next generation. Moreover, even as the social problems are being intensified and passed on, the means to deal with such a crisis is being taken away by irresponsible budgetary policies.

In December, 1989, former prosecutor and U.S. District Court Judge Robert Sweet, put it this way: "More money, more prisoners, more addicts-these numbers demonstrate to me our present prohibitive policy has failed, flatly and without serious question...Drugs have become an escape for those without a stake in society...Let's face that honestly and recognize that we must alter our society to eliminate, or at least substantially reduce, poverty."[6]

Put in the most general way, this society has an enormous underclass problem. This is the class with all the problems everyone is, more or less, aware of, even as the problems elicit no political response save to place more of these people in jail. The "drug crisis" is but one aspect of this problem and the "drug crisis" impacts all the way down the line, on the street, in the schools and within the family. Even as the drug crisis can be understood to be one facet of a long-term crisis in public health, so too it can be understood as being one facet of the long-term and long neglected American underclass problem.

(4) *There has been a continuing metamorphosis of crisis, both within the drug crisis per se and with social problems in general.*

Regarding the metamorphosis of crisis within the "drug crisis," remember how the crisis is continually being displaced without ever being solved. Eliminate one drug from the "crisis" ("PCP" or "crack"), and another comes along ("ice"); reduce the action in one city (Miami), and the action heats up in another (Los Angeles); shut down one street and the dealers simply move to another; arrest any number of dealers and the field is only cleared for many others.

Moreover, the drug crisis on the street and in the home becomes a judicial system crisis as arrests multiply beyond the ability of the system to deal with the numbers. Drugs are said to "cause" crime. What is overlooked is that violent offenders must be released early to make room for the increasing numbers of drug offenders put behind bars. In this way, as dangerous offenders pour out of prison to make room for newly-minted drug offenders, the law enforcement option could well be making the streets less safe than before the crackdown against drugs.

Furthermore, even as drugs cannot be said to "cause" crime or psychopathology, but rather are understood to interact with and maintain some other problematic condition, so too, regarding social problems, problematic drug usage has the same effect. The lack of medical care has already been mentioned. In addition, the problem of schools, of providing quality education, or even adequate education for underclass youths, the problem of malnutrition and lack of mental health care, all these aggravate the problem of drug abuse. In turn, the problem of drug abuse interacts to worsen the problems within the schools and communities.

The resultant intensification of the crisis, as each factor (the lack of health care, poor schools, chaotic communities, drug abuse) interacts with the other, produces exactly what we find today—steadily decaying school systems and neighborhoods, as well as the construction of a "lost generation" of underclass youths of whatever color and ethnicity.

(5) *The "war against drugs" has become a war against a people, primarily the people of the underclass but also the "counterculture."*

The "war against drugs" is innocently phrased by politicians, government officials and the statehouse press as a counterattack to all forms of drug use found within all socio-economic classes. But when we examine the execution of this policy, we find there is a particular population singled out, primarily the underclass, and that the problematic drug usage of mainstream America, alcohol and prescription drug abuse, is entirely ignored by public officials and even, in the case of tobacco, subsidized.

We do not find middle- and upper-class groups the objects of police action, as would be expected given that the drug crisis transcends class boundaries, that there are many times more middle-class individuals than individuals of the underclass, and that there exists, as a conservative estimate, a $100 billion illicit drug market. It is not possible for the underclass, given their income, to generate such a market. Such a market, produced by disposable income, must be largely fueled by middle- and upper- income groups. But we do not find these income groups the target of police action. Instead, the rise in arrests and imprisonment rates are drawn from the pool of people that have traditionally filled American prisons—the poor, the minorities, the uneducated; in other words, the underclass.

The "war against drugs," an ambiguous "war" against a problem without a center, against a complex underground market and a complex picture of usage, gravitates away from the usage of the middle and upper-income user and toward the traditional (and safer) object of police action—the underclass user. Simple answers and simple villains are demanded. These are supplied by the quite visible hand of government and press. Nowhere does the public, press, legal drug industry or political leaders see, or ever care to speak out against, the genuine cause of the crisis—themselves.

Consequently, the underclass in this crisis is twice victimized; by the emphasis on police action on the one hand and by the lack of health care on the other. The outcome of these factors, when combined with political and media leadership that prefers to promote hysteria rather than dispassionate analysis, is to produce a war against a people.

There is one other group that is the object of the war: the members (or perhaps, more accurately, the memory) of the counterculture; individuals who choose non-conventional and non-mainstream drugs as their drugs of choice. The violent upheavals of the sixties have left lasting resentments, including resentments against the counterculture that challenged the assumptions of the era. Widespread illicit use of marijuana began in that era. To decriminalize or legalize such a substance would be to accept the counterculture of the sixties, not something establishment and conservative figures such as a Mr. Reagan or a Mr. Bush can be expected to do.

The civil war of the 1960s continues, with continual attacks on the values of the era as though the sixties were last year and not more than twenty years ago. Current drug laws, and the refusal to change them to meet changing times, reflect, in part, the continuing effort to deny and reject the counterculture values of the era. It is no accident that the same Reagan/Bush administration that launched the current chapter of "the war against drugs" also strenuously opposed the values of environmentalism, energy conservation, civil rights and the social welfare programs that originated in the "sixties." The "war against drugs" has become first and foremost a war against the underclass, but the controversy of the sixties continues in the guise of a drug war.

This is consistent with the general rule; drug issues are symbolic of underlying cultural issues. Moreover, the issue is always the same what culture is to govern?

(6) *The equating of drugs with crime becomes a self-fulfilling prophesy when this is used to justify more police action and less drug treatment.*

Lacking treatment, there is no alternative save police action. Moreover, given that the police cannot generate positive change but only, and to a degree, suppress the worst symptoms of a lack of social health, this social policy ensures that both drugs and crime, considered separately or together, will continue to remain a problem.

The simple argument is often made that drug use leads to crime. This is made on the basis of studies that demonstrate high correlations between having a drug in one's bloodstream and being arrested. However, the correlation is easily demonstrated to be spurious. If it were true that drug use leads to crime, that a person ingests a drug and then, zombie-like, proceeds to commit a crime, then we would have middle- and upper-income individuals committing crimes and getting arrested at the same rate as underclass individuals. But that is not the case. The police station and jails are instead filled with the usual suspects, the poor, the uneducated and the minorities.

When no medical treatment is available, what other outcome is possible save eventual pickup by the police?

After a certain stay in jail, alternatively and perhaps progressively, local, county, then state imprisonment, as others are met with the same problem and greater knowledge of both the sources of drugs and illegal income, combined with, once again, no treatment for the addiction or dependency, what is possible save further perpetuation of the cycle?

This policy by default (for indeed it is a policy and no less a policy for not being made explicit by Washington politicians and bureaucrats), while it fattens the budgets of local and national police, makes just as little sense when looked at in strictly budgetary terms. It costs $35,000 to incarcerate one person for one year; it would be far cheaper in the long run to provide first-class (rather than token) drug treatment.

But police authorities, at both the local and Federal level (and given recent law, the military must now be considered a branch of law enforcement), are not going to support such facilities if it means a lessening of their take from the public treasury. Further, politicians routinely gain office by waving the bloody shirt of law and order and by promising to shut down the public welfare system (including public health programs). Media reports, written by the inexpert, tend to reflect back social biases as fact rather than to undercut and critically examine such biases. So no brakes are applied to the self-perpetuating and self-fulfilling prophesy that equates drugs with crime. Instead, yet more funding is proposed for law-enforcement and yet more arrests and more prisons are proposed by public officials.

Were no drug crisis to truly exist, such actions, when combined with the failure to fund health programs and then combined with the various hypocrisies of the law enforcement approach, would produce a drug crisis with all the features of the present one.

(7) *The more the law-enforcement option is pursued, the worse the crisis will become.*

To understand the "crisis," it is important to separate the primary effects of drug usage from the secondary effects, the effects of drug laws.

The effect of increasing law enforcement will probably be to weed out the lesser dealers and to clear the field for professional criminals, individuals who are simply not deterred by law enforcement. Further, the laws will only serve to further empower such individuals by maintaining their source of income and increasing the penalties will possibly increase the violence aimed against the police. In these ways, the law enforcement option will increase rather than alleviate the problem.

Court dockets and prisons are already full, indeed overflowing with drug offenders. Seeking to mitigate the crisis by pushing for more law enforcement will only worsen these problems. Then there is the problem of the diminution of constitutional protections, of the enhancement of governmental and police authority at the expense of individual liberty—this is more likely to be the enduring legacy of the "war against drugs," rather than any diminution of either drug usage or crime.

In addition, there is the problem of official corruption, of "honest citizen" and "upstanding citizen" type criminal activity. These problems will continue as the drug war continues. Referring to the latter, the cash flow of the drug trade is enormous and will continue to tempt individuals who are otherwise law-abiding and responsible citizens. The longer present policy continues, the longer there will be a greater number of such individuals, to the social detriment of all. Such policies are as responsible for the drug crisis as the pharmacological and social-psychological effects of any particular drug.

(8) *The "drug crisis," in all its aspects, is not the outcome of drug usage; the crisis is caused by bad law.*

It is bad law that fills the courts and prisons with problems that are primarily a question of health care rather than criminal activity and bad law that overlooks the practices of the well-connected while focusing on the disempowered. It is bad law that reduces rather than preserves individual liberty. It is bad law that treats social problems as simply a problem of crime, overlooking the fundamental sources of the problem simply for the expediency of re-election concerns. It is bad law that seeks to enforce a rigid stance on a society that is multicultural (and is so quite apart from ethnicities per se). Indeed, the fact that the Federal government itself ignores its own "war against drugs" is the critical evidence of the shallowness of the "war" and the hollow nature of current law.

How can such law and such facts as presented here be accounted for, referring now to all the facts of the "drug crisis?" Following interpretations that can be found in the various writings of Arnold Trebach, Ethan Nadelmann, as well as Samuel Eliot Morrison, the argument here is that such laws and policies are the outcome of larger social facts and not any sort of weighing of pharmacological or psychological risk. The drug preferences of the middle-class and upper income groups, plus the traditional disdain for the underclass and the political influence of the alcohol and tobacco manufacturers: these are the facts that can explain the ambiguities and contradictions of current law and policies.

(9) *Laws that disregard the relevant social facts of the larger society are doomed to failure. Worse yet, they are bound to exacerbate rather than mitigate the problem the laws are ostensibly meant to address. To effectively meet the American drug problem, laws must be drawn that consider the larger social milieu, and then action must be taken directly within that larger milieu, rather than relying solely on law and law enforcement.*

Still, once complete legalization is rejected, the question remains: how might drug laws be drawn and what sort of thinking should guide their construction?

Boiling down the problem confronting social policy and the drug crisis to its simplest form: on one hand, there is the problem of the potential increase in numbers of addicted and problematic users were drug laws liberalized, while on the other hand, there is the problem of the underground market, of empowering career criminals, if the drug laws are not liberalized.

In other words, the problem is to minimize the following: to minimize addiction, to minimize the social harm the addicted (or more generally, those who fail to exercise self-control) can cause others, and to minimize the empowerment handed career criminals by laws that construct an underground market. No simple thing, not something that can be done via the application of mechanistic formulas.

As individual initiative and sensibility have been the prime mitigators of the problem of usage, the aim of policy should be to strengthen individual initiative and equally, to discourage (at least not encourage) drug-taking in whatever form. An implicit theme of the current hysteria is that drugs are powerful but people are not. This is just the wrong message to give. People are powerful; drugs are not.

Further, demonizing substances only serves to give them a mystique that, however paradoxically, encourages usage. One example of demonization encouraging negative behavior is the emulation by middle-class youths of "gangs." A second proof of the power of mystique is the Dutch example, where a straightforward and demystifying approach to marijuana has created usage rates that are one-tenth the American rate.

A sensible way to cut through the problem is simply to establish priorities, like the Dutch. Second, policies should be consistent with each other. Last, such policies should be consistent with the larger society, the multicultural, multidimensional post-modern world. The following recommendations regarding the five prime drugs of concern—tobacco, alcohol, marijuana, cocaine and heroin—were formed within this context.

(A) Tobacco: Present social policy is to subsidize tobacco growers while, on the other hand, taxing tobacco sales to provide funding for any number of public services.

It makes no sense to subsidize the growing of tobacco. Supposedly, we do live in a system in which the "invisible hand" of the market determines sales rather than the very visible hand of government subsidies. Moreover, government subsidies of a drug responsible for one thousand deaths a day is beyond reason, save that reason itself rarely guides public policymaking. The cause of such subsidies is equally obvious—the political influence of the tobacco lobby. This is an example of how our drug policies are created by the application of such influence, rather than by considerations of public health.

Nonetheless, the sensible public policy would end such subsidies and greatly increase the taxing of tobacco to provide the funding for drug treatment and education programs, as well as for mental health clinics and subsidies of emergency rooms.

(B) Alcohol: Alcohol is available not because it is safe, alcohol is available because prohibition failed. Present social policy is to allow unlimited promotions of such drugs, even though purchase of the drug is restricted. Such promotions should be banned.

Certainly, a social policy based on truly engaging the drug crisis, instead of a social policy based on not offending the alcohol lobby, would end the promotion of alcohol sales on television. The banning of cigarette ads and the subsequent decline in tobacco use is a demonstration of the effectiveness of such a measure. The decline of tobacco usage is the greatest success story in the history of "what worked." The success could well be duplicated in the other mainstream drug of choice. The difficulty here is the political influence of the alcohol lobby and its influence in the television and print industry, for whom alcohol ads are a lucrative revenue.

The unlimited promotion of alcohol is senseless, if public health and the health of young people were a priority of social policy. A further recommendation is to increase alcohol taxes to provide for treatment and health programs of the kind recommended above.

(C) Marijuana: No drug is "safe." Safety is a relative thing: relative to alcohol and tobacco, marijuana is a far safer drug of choice. The present prohibition makes no sense and, indeed, unofficial policy and the decriminalization of marijuana in a number of states recognizes this. In states that have decriminalized marijuana, the increases that have occurred have been no greater than in states that did not decriminalize. For the Dutch, decriminalization of marijuana has not resulted in an explosion of usage; on the contrary, usage rates for Dutch youth is one-tenth the usage rates for American youth.

The general rule is that increased availability leads to increased usage, however, in the case of decriminalization, that increased usage appears to be constrained. The recommendation is to make the drug laws consistent with one another and to decriminalize marijuana.

An argument could be made for legalization. Legalization could be limited to, more or less, present custom and restricted to private use within the home. The taxes generated by sales could then be used to support the health programs noted above. However, there are two obstacles to such legalization. First, there are the international agreements that have been signed with regard to domestic drug laws and second, there is considerable opposition at home to such a policy. Moreover, such opposition has a core of research fact to support it, given the general rule that increased availability leads to increased usage.

This opposition includes opposition to decriminalization. What must be appreciated is that alcohol prohibition failed not because alcohol consumption remained stable or increased during the prohibition years, in fact, consumption declined. Prohibition "failed" in that the negative consequences of the policy were recognized and, eventually, dealt with by ending the badly conceived law. As for marijuana we are dealing with a prohibition problem that is of a lesser degree, simply because fewer people use the drug. Nonetheless, given the amounts of money generated by the present prohibition, particularly when cocaine is included, the failure is just as great and the consequences are just as great (referring to police and official corruption, as well as "honest citizen" and "upstanding citizen" type crime). That failure needs to be recognized.

Even if decriminalization of marijuana is thought too radical, the dispensing of marijuana for legitimate medical purposes should be permitted. Two prime uses of marijuana are for the treatment of glaucoma and as an adjunct to cancer chemotherapy. Marijuana relieves the constant nausea and vomiting that are an unfortunate and inevitable side effect of cancer medication. Indeed, in a recent informal poll, some 48 percent of cancer specialists reported they would prescribe marijuana in such cases were it legal to do so.[7]

According to the prime source used above, the *Encyclopedia Britannica,* marijuana may also be useful in the treatment of depression, loss of appetite, high blood pressure, anxiety, migraine, and for a number of gynecological and menstrual problems. Of course, this does not mean marijuana is a "health" drug and, as true of all drugs, usage can lead to the abuse problems of dependency, avoidance behavior, and various physical ailments. In the case of marijuana, the clearest problem concerning physical harm is that of lung damage.

Current policy opposing prescription use makes little sense. For example, under current law it is perfectly legal to prescribe morphine for cancer patients but not marijuana. The U.S. Court of Appeals, responding to reports of the plant's medical uses, has ordered the DEA to reconsider its marijuana policy. Moreover, the DEA's own administrative judge has recommended that marijuana be permitted as a prescription drug, only to be overruled by top-level officials.[8]

The hemp plant may have commercial and environmental value as well. According to a number of writers, the hemp plant produces four times more paper pulp per acre than wood pulp. Further, hemp paper is used as the material of English and Canadian banknotes because the paper lasts considerably longer than paper made from wood pulp. Hence, the hemp plant has the potential to be an important environmental tool, given the continuing controversy over how best to protect our nation's, and the world's, forests.[9]

(D) Cocaine: This is the most problematic of drugs to regulate. The cocaine fad of the late 1890s ended when the negative effects of the drug became widely known (a good example of the effectiveness of drug education) and when the drug lost its "elite" image and gained an underclass image. However, from our own history, there is also an example of the failure of education and prohibition, meaning alcohol prohibition.

The critical question is this: is cocaine usage in our time like the earlier "fad" and bound to end or is cocaine usage now like alcohol usage? Meaning, even with its negative effects known and even given a prohibition, demand is so insistent as to overwhelm efforts at social control. The further problem, of course, is that proposals of regulation must be based on the true facts of the crisis of usage and these facts, as seen, are quite unclear.

Quite likely, no sort of regulation is truly going to work. Cocaine usage rates are likely to remain at historical highs, with recent declines bottoming out at rates that, though lower than the peak, remain higher than any previous period of time. The most sensible policy is probably to continue the present prohibition. The effects of marijuana decriminalization would permit a focusing on drugs such as cocaine with, presumably, greater enforcement effect.

It is also recommended that the law enforcement effort be redirected. There are two useful approaches yet to be tried in regard to the cocaine trade: immunity for the Colombian cartel leaders and "following the money."

Colombian cartel leaders have offered to cease their participation in the drug trade in exchange for amnesty. Their offer should be accepted. These individuals are energetic and talented businessmen who have constructed and maintained any number of international corporations. Much is to be gained, by both Colombia and the United States, by directing this energy and talent away from the drug trade and toward the legal market. Were they to break the agreement, law enforcement could be reapplied— and the more aboveground their businesses are, the more effectively could that enforcement be applied. Further, we need only consider the American lack of moral purity, referring to the nineteenth century importation of opium into China and the CIA's current involvement in the drug trade, to appreciate that the United States government is hard pressed to reject immunity in the name of morality.

Even if this is done, others, hopefully less organized and talented, will step into the cocaine trade. How can they be restrained?

The law enforcement policy here is to "follow the money." The trade generates an enormous amount of cash that must, to be spent, eventually end up in legitimate banks. This money market is a smaller market than the drug market and the technology and some of the laws necessary to track large sums of money are already in place. The one drawback has been the Reagan and Bush administrations' refusal to toughen reporting laws. Such refusal plays into the hands of the druglords.

(E) Heroin: From the research, only long-term methadone maintenance offers any sort of consistent success for heroin addiction. Success means problem management (and the problem heroin users can cause others via the property crimes committed to support the addiction) more than an absolute end to addiction. The problem is that such programs are being short-changed in the general hysteria and promotion of the law-enforcement option.

Furthermore, the very character of the population reduces the possibility of giving help. For example, the poor outcome of needle exchange programs, evidently because of suspicions regarding arrest, and the finding that the sharing of needles (of course, a leading cause of AIDS) is considered an act of friendship between addicts, discourage one from proposing liberal solutions. Still, apparently the best policy is the Dutch policy of limiting the damage and social harm such individuals can cause others. This is the one policy that has reduced the numbers of addicts (outside of Singapore—whose policy is the death penalty for sellers). Moreover, the Dutch approach has made it possible to gain an accurate count of the number of addicted. This is not to say that America would want to import the whole Dutch policy. However, treatment on demand, including needle exchange, appears to be a policy superior to our own.

The comparative literature on heroin treatment in Britain and the United States is as tangled a literature as there is in the field of drug policy. No approach is without controversy within its own borders and this includes the Dutch approach. There appears to be good reason for this; nothing works, unless a relative standard is applied. There are only hard choices, none of which are particularly defensible, as opponents can always find ample evidence of failure. The three countries noted here thereby tend to settle into the approach consistent with their larger cultural understandings; the Dutch into a liberal social laissez-faire, the English placing treatment within the privileged relationship accorded the doctor and patient, and the United States trusting to law-enforcement.

Though no approach works well enough to be non-controversial, nonetheless, this is a poor defense for the non-policy of the United States. Americans have opted for a law enforcement approach to heroin addiction, but this policy is not the outcome of deliberate debate and decision as much as the inevitable result of the consistent rejection of the health and treatment approach. In other words, current policy is the outcome of a paralysis of policy and a policy by default, not of a rational weighing of costs and benefits. Americans insist on a moral definition of the problem and hence any pragmatic policy that seeks to make the hard choices becomes open to bloody shirt arguments, to the charge of encouraging usage or coddling the morally bankrupt.

The first priority must be prevention. Prevention begins with interdiction, the rejection of cooperation with the underground market (referring to the CIA and DEA overseas operations), and a close supervision of hospital supplies. Treatment on demand, the registration of addicts in exchange for methadone maintenance, and then needle exchange programs to reduce the volume of AIDS cases (and hence the likelihood of the infection of others via blood supplies), all appear commonsensical even if controversial. The purpose is to minimize the harm the addict can cause the general public.

What can be said of a country with an enormous underclass problem that decides to handle the problem by spending more money on law enforcement and by expanding available prison space? Certainly this question appears between the lines here and therefore, in conclusion, is worth examining explicitly.

There are two truths to America relevant to the argument presented here. First of all, America is a land with a history of great injustices. There is the history of slavery, a history that stained the democratic experiment from its first days. Moreover, the discrimination faced by Chinese Americans, particularly in the nineteenth century, and the discrimination against Japanese Americans, especially the taking away of all they owned and their incarceration in internment camps during World War II, and the discrimination that continues against Latino Americans and Americans of color are all instances in a history of injustice.

The one comfort that might be drawn here is that few Americans have escaped such prejudice and discrimination. The Italian, the Irish and the Jew of the early twentieth century all faced the same sort of discrimination. Further, were we to yet broaden our focus, we would find, for example, German Americans undergoing the same sort of thing in the eighteenth century. Few have escaped the injustice of prejudice and discrimination.

Perhaps it is the poverty of a group that inspires discrimination, as well as the seeming permission to practice discrimination and prejudice, rather than color or language or religion or any other sort of difference. Whatever the case, the fact remains, the history of America is a history of injustice against particular groups at particular points in time, with, no doubt, people of color and the people of that era's underclass being doubly victimized.

But then there is a second truth: America remains a land of great opportunity. Opportunity is here defined as the opportunity to make one's own opportunity. Such a statement is so often made by politicians that it is a cliche. Yet "opportunity" remains a fact supported by research. In America, 1 in 10 individuals who had working-class fathers reach the professional class. This may sound alarming (though, of course, it ignores the numbers of people who did not attempt such a jump). However, consider the statistics from other countries: in Japan, 1 in 14 make the leap, 1 Swede in 50, 1 Frenchman in 67, 1 Dane in 100, 1 Italian in 300.[10] What can account for the greater social mobility in the United States?

Generally, experts agree that the enhanced potential for social mobility here is due to an open educational system. For those who finish high school (regretfully, our dropout rates are the highest in the developed world), there is a college nearby with an open enrollment commitment, quite possibly within commuting distance. That is a tribute to our dedication to higher education. Whatever is wrong with the American system of education, there have also been successes.

The proposal is that a second pillar be added to the American commitment to social mobility—a public health system. How is it that we can minimize the consequences of past discrimination and injustice and enhance the America of great opportunity? A public health system in which no American would do without the benefits of health care would be the single most effective measure we could undertake to enhance the best side of our society. Individuals who grow up without health care are placed at an enormous disadvantage vis à vis others.

Moreover, as previously stated, such individuals are deprived of a basic advantage to being an American, access to the best medicine in the world, while on the other hand, they are burdened by the injustice of a police and judicial system that focuses on controlling the underclass. Access to health care is as precious as access to the ballot box.

By health care via a public health system is meant first and foremost, universal health insurance. Also included are mental health care and drug treatment programs as well as a full range of health information programs, distributed via the television and radio media. In addition, an emergency care network should be funded so that no person would be further than 20 minutes from the nearest health care facility. There also would be an expanded national health center that is empowered to be proactive toward health crises. Some may claim this is a "wish list." The fact is we are the only modern nation without such a system.

Returning to the drug crisis, there are many faces and locations for the crisis in usage and many different sorts of crises that could be focused on other than usage. But to a large extent there is only one crisis: the crisis in health care delivery. Until universal health care is extended to the underclass, we will produce unending crises to either overlook or to sloganize.

The Victorian stance governs in our time. This stance claims the crisis is a problem of values, a problem families are having rather than a problem a society is having. This is not unreasonable but it blinds proponents to the larger origin of the problem—the society that produced the crisis.

Hence, the social-level influence of, for example, alcohol advertising, is entirely ignored. Moreover, the Victorian stance is a moralistic stance: people simply should not do such and such a behavior. The moralistic stance favors the law enforcement approach as the appropriate recourse when the frowned-upon behavior continues.

Such a perspective, rejecting social-level analysis, leads to the rejection of social-level action, such as the building of a first-rate public health system. Hence police action becomes social policy by default. The outcome is poor social policy and ineffective police action. A further problem of the moral stance is that it is not backed by a moral commitment to the health and welfare of the nation's youth. Rather, the moral stance serves as a cover for the denial and rationalization of the inconvenient truth. The mindset, the very frame of understanding, perpetuates the crisis.

We created the crisis not, as conventionally put, the pharmacological properties of some drug. The goal of this work was to thoroughly analyze the crisis and to make explicit and obvious how this is so.

Notes

1. "Did Cocaine Sting Fuel Drug Sales?," *Los Angeles Times,* 14 June 1989.
2. "F.A.A. Faulted Over Crew That Drank," *New York Times,* 13 March 1990.
3. "U.S. Report Raises Estimate of Smoking Toll," *New York Times,* 11 January 1989.
4. "Short Supplies May Be Diluting Street Cocaine," *Los Angeles Times,* 22 May 1990. See also "Coca Price Collapse Offers Opportunity in Drug War," *Los Angeles Times,* 21 May 1990.
5. Peter Reuter, *Sealing the Borders.*
6. U.S. Judge Calls for Legalization of Illicit Drugs," *Washington Post,* 13 December 1989. See also "Nothing Else Has Worked: Abolish the Prohibitions," Los Angeles Times, 12 March 1990. This opinion piece was by Judge Sweet.
7. "48% of Cancer Specialists in Study Would Prescribe Pot," *Los Angeles Times,* 1 May 1991.
8. Jack Herer, *The Emperor Wears No Clothes,* (Van Nuys, CA: HEMP, 1990). The work is the most enthusiastic (and fact-filled) I have read in favor of the hemp plant and its legalization.
9. Ibid.
10. Ian Robertson, *Sociology,* 3rd ed. (New York: Worth Publications, 1987), 276. Also, for a history of this aspect of American history, a standard work is Daniel Boorstein's *The Americans: the Democratic Experience* (New York: Random House, 1973). For a history that presents America in its fullest complexity, a standard work is Samuel Eliot Morrison's *The Oxford History of the American People* (New York: Oxford University Press, 1965).

References

Able, Ernest L., and Phillip Zeidenberg. "Alcohol and Homicide: A Comparison between Erie County, New York and Los Angeles County, California." *American Journal of Drug and Alcohol Abuse* 12(1986): 121-29.

Alfred Lindesmith. *The Addict and the Law.* Bloomington: Indiana University Press, 1965.

American Academic Encyclopedia. Danbury, CT: Grolier, 1990.

Anglen, Douglas M., and Yih-Ing Hsu. "Treatment of Drug Abuse." In *Drugs and Crime,* edited by James Q. Wilson and Michael Toney. Chicago: University of Chicago Press, 1990.

Barnes, Deborah. "Breaking the Cycle of Addiction." *Science* 241(1988): 1029-30.

Barsky, Arthur J. "The Paradox of Health." *New England Journal of Medicine* 318(7)(1988): 414-18.

Becker, Howard. *The Outsiders. London:* The Free Press, 1963.

Bell, Daniel. *The Coming of the Post-Industrial Society.* New York: Basic Books, 1973.

Berk, Richard. "Causal Inference in the Social Sciences." In *Handbook of Sociology,* edited by Neil Smelser. Newbury Park, CA: Sage Publications, 1988.

Berkeley, Edmund C. *The Computer Revolution.* Garden City, NY: Doubleday, 1962.

Black, Claudia. *It Will Never Happen To Me.* Denver: M.A.C., 1981.

Blum, Richard. *Drug Education: Results and Recommendations.* Lexington, MA: Lexington Books, 1976.

Board of Trustees Report, American Medical Association. "Alcohol: Advertising, Counteradvertising and Depiction in the Media." *Journal of the American Medical Association* 256(11)(1986): 1485-88.

Boorstein, Daniel. *The Americans: The Democratic Experience.* New York: Random House, 1973.

Brady, Rosemary. "In Dutch." *Forbes,* 27 February 1984, 46.

Brown, Larry J. "Hunger in the U.S." *Scientific American, February* 1987, 37-41

Brown, Stephanie. *Treating Adult Children of Alcoholics: A Developmental Perspective.* New York: Wiley, 1988.

Buckley, William E., Charles E. Yesalis, Karl E. Friedl, William A. Anderson, Andrea L. Streit, and James E. Wright. "Estimated Prevalence of Anabolic Steroid Use among Male High School Seniors." *Journal of the American Medical Association* 260(23)(1988): 3441-45.

Budd, Robert D. "Cocaine Abuse and Violent Death." *American Journal of Drug and Alcohol Abuse*, 15(4)(1989): 375-82.

Budiansky, Stephen. "A Measure of Failure." *Atlantic Monthly*, January 1986, 32-34.

Caper, Philip. "Solving the Medical Care Dilemma." *New England Journal of Medicine* 318(23)(1988): 1535-36.

Centers for Disease Control. *Alcohol and Fatal Injuries—Fulton County, Georgia, 1982.* Morbidity and Mortality Weekly Reports 1983, 32: 573-76.

Cermak, Timmen. *Primer for Adult Children of Alcoholics.* Pompano Beach, FL: Health Communications, 1985.

Chambliss, William. "The Political Economy of Smack: Opiates, Capitalism and Law." *Research in Law and Sociology* 1(1978): 115-41.

Clayton, Richard, Harwin L. Voss, Cynthia Robbins, and William Skinner. "Gender Differences in Drug Use: An Epidemiological Perspective." In *Women and Drugs: A New Era for Research.* National Institute of Drug Abuse Research Monograph #65. Washington, DC: U.S. Government Printing Office, 1986.

Cloninger, Robert, Michael Bohman, and Soren Sigvardson. "Inheritance of Alcohol Abuse." *Archives of General Psychiatry* 38(1981): 861-68.

Cockburn, Leslie. Out of Control: The Story of the Reagan Administration's Secret War in Nicaragua, the Illegal Arms Pipeline, and the Contra Drug Connection. New York: The Atlantic Monthly Press, 1987.

Collins, James J., ed. *Drinking and Crime: Perspectives on the Relationship between Alcohol and Criminal Behavior.* New York: Guilford Press, 1981.

Covington, Stephanie S., and Janet Kohen. "Women, Alcohol and Sexuality." *Advances in Alcohol and Substance Abuse* 4(1)(1984): 41-56.

Davis, Wade. *Passage of Darkness: The Ethnobiology of the Haitian Zombie.* Chapel Hill: The University of North Carolina Press, 1988.

Dean, Malcolm. "The Dutch Soft-Drug Policy." *Lancet,* 21 October 1989, 993-94

Destouzas, Michael L., and Joel Moses. *The Computer Age: A Twenty-year View.* Cambridge, MA: M.I.T. Press, 1979.

Duster, Troy. *The Legislation of Morality.* New York: Free Press, 1970.

The New Encyclopedia Britannica, Micropedia, 15th Edition. Chicago: Encyclopedia Britannica, Inc., 1974.

Etizoni, Amitri. *The Active Society.* New York: The Free Press, 1968.

Forbes, David. "Saying No to Ron and Nancy: School-Based Drug Abuse Prevention Programs in the 1980s." *Journal of Education* 169(3)(1987): 80-90.

Frieze, Irene H., and Patricia C. Schafer. "Alcohol Use and Marital Violence: Female and Male Differences in Reactions to Alcohol." In *Alcohol Problems in Women: Antecedents, Consequences and Intervention,* edited by Sharon C. Wilsnack and Linda J. Beckman. New York: Guilford Press, 1984.

The Gallup Poll Monthly. "Widespread Opposition to Drug Legalization," 292 (January 1990): 2-8.

——-. "Keys to Fighting Drugs Seen as Educating Youth, Halting Supply." 270 (March 1988): 32-33.

Gerson, Lowell W., and Donald A. Preston. "Alcohol Consumption and the Incidence of Violent Crime." *Journal of Studies of Alcohol* 40: (March 1979): 307-12.

Gillman, Cherni. "New York City's Needle Exchange Experiment: Policy Implications From It's First Year." In *Problems of Drug Dependence 1990: Proceedings of the 52nd Annual Scientific Meeting of the Committee on Problems of Drug Dependence.* Research Monograph No. 105. Washington, DC: Government Printing Office, 1990.

Glassner, Barry and Bruce Berg. "How Jews Avoid Alcohol Problems." *American Sociological Review* 45(1980): 647-64.

Gleiberman, Lillian, Ernest Harburg, Wayne Di Franceisco, and Anthony Schork. "Familial Transmission of Alcoholism." *International Journal of Epidemiology* 20(2)(1991): 441-47.

Goodwin, Donald W., Fini Schulsinger, Leif Hermansen, Samuel B. Guze, and George Winokur. "Alcohol Problems in Adoptees Raised Apart from Alcoholic Biological Parents." *Archives of General Psychiatry* 28(1973): 238-43.

Grady, Katherine, Kelin E. Gersick, David L. Snow, and Marion Kessen. "The Emergence of Adolescent Substance Abuse." *Journal of Drug Education* 16(3)(1986): 203-19.

Gravitz, Herbert, and Julie Bowden. *Theraputic Issues of Adult Children of Alcoholics.* Holmes Beach, FL: Learning Publications, 1985.

Gropper, Bernard. "Probing the Links between Drugs and Crime." In *National Institute of Justice: Research in Brief.* Washington, DC: National Institute of Justice, 1985.

Haberman, Paul, and Michael Baden. *Alcohol, Other Drugs and Violent Death.* New York: Oxford University Press, 1978.

Harris, Louis. *Inside America.* New York: Vintage, 1987.

Hayashida, Motoi, Arthur I. Alterman, A. Thomas McCellan, Charles P. O'Brien, James Purtell, Joseph R. Volpicelli, Arnold H. Raphaelson, and Charles P. Hall. "Comparative Effectiveness and Costs of Inpatient and Outpatient Detoxification of Patients with Mild-to-Moderate Alcohol Withdrawal Syndrome." *New England Journal of Medicine* 320(6)(1989): 358-65.

Helvey, T.C. *The Age of Information: An Interdisciplinary Survey of Cybernetics.* Englewood Cliffs, NJ: Educational Technology Publications, 1971.

Hendin, Herbert, and Ann Pollinger Haas. "The Adaptive Significance of Chronic Marijuana Use for Adolescents and Adults." *Advances in Alcohol and Drug Abuse* 4(3/4)(1985): 99-115.

Herbert, J. Gans. *The Urban Villagers.* Glencoe: The Free Press, 1962.

Herer, Jack. *The Emperor Wears No Clothes.* Van Nuys, CA: HEMP, 1990.

Hoadley, John F., Beth C. Fuchs, and Harold D. Holder. "The Effect of Alcohol Beverage Restrictions on Consumption: A 25-year Longitudinal Analysis." *American Journal of Drug and Alcohol Abuse.* 10(3)(1984): 375-401.

Hoffman, Abbie. "Reefer Madness." *The Nation,* 21 November 1987, 580.

Holden, Constance. "Is Alcohol Treatment Effective?" *Science* 236(1987): 20-22.

Holsten, Fred. "The Female Drug Abuser: Has She a Shorter Way Out?" *The Journal of Drug Issues* 15(3)(1985): 383-92.

Hundley, John D. "Drug Usage and Outstanding Performance Among Young Adolescents." *Addictive Behaviors* 10(1985): 419-23.

Huxley, Aldous. *The Doors of Perception.* New York: Harper & Row, 1954.

Inciardi, James, ed. *The Drug Legalization Debate.* Newbury Park, CA: Sage Publications, 1991.

Inciardi, James. *War on Drugs: Heroin, Cocaine, Crime and Public Policy.* Palo Alto, CA: Mayfield Press, 1986.

Inter-University Consortium for Political and Social Research. *ABC News Drug Abuse Poll,* 1986. 1988. ICPSR 8636.Ann Arbor, MI: ICPSR.

Jackson, Joan. "The Adjustment of the Family to the Crisis of Alcoholism." *Quarterly Journal of Studies of Alcoholism* 15(1954): 562-86.

Jacobs, James B. "Drinking and Crime." In *National Institute of Justice Crime File Series.* Washington, DC: National Institute of Justice, 1984.

Johnston, L. Testimony delivered at hearings on the effects of marijuana, Senate subcommittee on Criminal Justice, Judiciary Committee, 16 January, 1980.

Jones, Helen C., and Paul W. Lovinger. *The Marijuana Question.* New York: Dodd Mead, 1985.

Kaufman, Edward. "The Relationship of Social Class and Ethnicity to Drug Abuse." In *A Multicultural View of Drug Abuse,* edited by David Smith. Cambridge, MA: Schenkman, 1985.

Kirn, Timothy F. "Drug Abuse: More Help Available for Addicted Persons but Main Problem Continues Unabated." *Journal of the American Medical Association,* 260(15) (1988): 2170-72.

Klassen, Albert, Colin J. Williams, and Eugene E. Levitt. In *Sex and Morality in the U.S.: An Empirical Study under the Auspices of the Kinsey Institute.* Middletown, CT: Wesleyan University Press, 1989.

Kwitny, Jonathan. *Crimes of Patriots: A True Tale of Dope, Dirty Money and the CIA.* New York: W. W. Norton, 1987.

Lang, Alan R. "The Social Psychology of Drinking and Human Sexuality." *Journal of Drug Issues* 15(2)(1985): 273-89.

Leigh, Barbara C. "Beliefs about the Effects of Alcohol on Self and Others." *Journal of Studies on Alcohol* 48(5)(1987): 467-75.

———. "The Powers of John Barleycorn: Beliefs about the Effects of Alcohol on Social Behavior." *American Psychologist* 41(1986): 751-64.

Letteri, Dan J. "Drug Abuse: A Review of Explanations and Models of Explanation." *Advances in Alcohol and Substance Abuse* 4(3/4)(1985): 9-23.

Lindesmith, Alfred. *The Addict and the Law.* Bloomington: Indiana University Press, 1965.

Macdonald, T. Patrick, and Rhoda Estep. "Prime Time Drug Depictions." *Contemporary Drug Problems* 12(3)(1985): 419-30.

Macdonald, Scott B. *Dancing on a Volcano: The Latin-American Drug*

Trade. New York: Praeger, 1988.

Maloff, Deborah. "A Review of the Effects of the Decriminalization of Marijuana." *Contemporary Drug Problems* 10(3)(1981): 307-21.

Marlatt, G. Alan, and Judith R. Gordon, eds. *Relapse Prevention.* New York: Guilford Press, 1985.

Marshall, Eliot. "The Drug of Champions." *Science* 242 (1988): 183-84.

———. "Legalization Gets a Hearing." *Science* 241 (1988): 1157-59.

———. "A War on Drugs with Real Troops?" *Science* 241 (1988): 13-15.

Mauer, Mark. *Young Black Men and the Criminal Justice System: A Growing National Problem.* Washington, DC: The Sentencing Project, 1990.

Mayer, Joseph, and Rebecca Black. "Relationship between Alcoholism and Child Abuse and Neglect." In *Currents in Alcoholism,* vol. 2, edited by Frank A. Sexius. New York: Grune and Stratton, 1977.

McCoy, Alfred E., Cathleen B. Read, and Leonard P. Adams, II. *The Politics of Heroin in Southeast Asia.* New York: Harper & Row, 1972.

McLuhan, Marshall, and Bruce R. Powers. *The Global Village: Transformations in World Life and Media in the 21st Century.* New York: Oxford University Press, 1989.

Miller, William R., and Nick Heather. *Treating Addictive Behavior: Process of Change.* New York: Plenum Press, 1986.

Millman, Joel. "Narco-terroism: A tale of two stories." *Columbian Journalism Review* 25(1986): 48-51.

Moore, Richard D., Lee R. Bone, Gail Geller, Joyce Marnon, Emma J. Stokes, and David M. Levine. "Prevalence, Detection and Treatment of Alcoholism in Hospitalized Patients." *Journal of the American Medical Association* 261(3)(1989): 403-8.

Morley, Jefferson. "The Kid Who Sold Crack to the President." *Washington City Paper,* 15-21 December 1989.

Morrison, Samuel Eliot. *Oxford History of the American People.* New York: Oxford University Press, 1965.

Musto, David. *The American Disease,* 2d ed. New Haven: Yale University Press, 1987.

Nadalmann, Ethan A. "U.S. Drug Policy: A Bad Export." *Foreign Policy* 70 (1988): 83-108.

Nadelmann, Ethan A. "The Case for Legalization." *Public Interest* 92 (Summer 1988): 3-31.

National Institute of Alcohol Abuse and Alcoholism (NIAAA). *Sixth Special Report to the U.S. Congress on Alcohol and Health.* DHHS Pub. No. (ADM) 97-1519. Washington, DC: U.S. Government Printing Office, 1987.

National Institute of Drug Abuse (NIDA). *Drug Use among American High School Students, College Students and Other Young Adults—National Trends through 1989.* Washington, DC: U.S. Government Printing Office, 1989.

———. *Drug Use among High School Students, College Students, and Other Young Adults—National Trends through 1988.* Washington, DC: U.S. Government Printing Office, 1988.

Newcomb, Michael D. and Peter Bentley. *Consequences of Adolescent*

Drug Use: Impact on the Lives of Young Adults. Newbury Park, CA: Sage, 1988.

Newsweek. "Uncivil Liberties?" 23 April 1990, 18-20.

———. "The Alcohol Gender Gap," 22 January 1990, 53.

———. "Taking on the Legalizers," 25 December 1989, 46.

———. "A DEA Hero is Busted," 28 August 1989, 32.

———. "Forgotten Patients," 22 August 1989, 52-53.

———. "Southwest Connection," 23 November 1987, 29-33.

———. "Trauma in the Emergency Room," 16 February 1987, 76-77.

———. "The Friends of David T," 10 February 1986, 68.

Pentz, Mary Ann, James H. Dwyer, David P. Mackinnon, Brian R. Flay, William B. Hansen, Eric Yu. I. Wang, and C. Anderson Johnson. "A Multicommunity Trial for Primary Prevention of Adolescent Drug Abuse." *Journal of the American Medical Association* 261(22)(1989): 3259-66.

Pratt, William F., and Christine A. Bachrach. "What Do Women Use When They Stop Using the Pill?" *Family Planning Perspectives* 19(6)(1987): 257-66.

Reuter, Peter, Gordon Crawford, and Jonathan Cave. *Sealing the Borders.* R-3594-USDP. Washington, DC: RAND National Defense Research Institute, 1988.

Reuter, Peter, John Haaga, Patrick Murphy, and Amy Praskac. *Drug Use and Drug Programs in the Washington Metropolitan Area.* R-3655-GWRC. Santa Monica: RAND Corporation, 1988.

Reuter, Peter, Robert Maccoum, and Patrick Murphy. *Money from Crime: The Economics of Drug Dealing in Washington, DC* R-3894-RF. Santa Monica: RAND Corporation, 1990.

Riesman, David. *The Lonely Crowd.* New Haven: Yale University Press, 1950.

Robertson, Ian. *Sociology,* 3d ed. New York: Worth Publications, 1987.

Room, Robin. *Alcohol and Disinhibition: Nature and Meaning of the Link,* Research Monograph No. 12. Report of a conference held 11-13 February 1981, Berkeley, CA.

Rouse, John Jay, and Bruce D. Johnson. "Hidden Paradigms of Morality in Debates About Drugs: Historical and Policy Shifts in British and American Drug Policy." In *The Drug Legalization Debate,* edited by James Inciardi. Newbury Park, CA: Sage Publications, 1991.

Russell, Bertrand. *Mysticism and Logic.* New York: W. W. Norton, 1929.

Russell, Marcia, Cynthia Henderson, and Sheila B. Blume. *Children of Alcoholics: A Review of the Literature.* Buffalo: New York State Division of Alcoholism and Alcohol Abuse, Research Institute on Alcoholism, 1985.

Schaps, Eric, Joel M. Moskowitz, Janet H. Malvin, and Gary A. Schaeffer. "Evaluation of Seven School-based Prevention Programs: A Final Report on the Napa Project." *International Journal of the Addictions* 21(1986): 1081-112.

Schuckit, Marc A. "Alcoholism and Affective Disorders: Diagnostic Confusion." In *Alcohol and Dependency,* edited by D.W. Goodwin. New York: Spectrum, 1984.

Schur, Edwin. *Narcotics in Britain and the U.S.* Bloomington: Indiana

University Press, 1962.

Siegel, Ronald K. "Cocaine and the Priviledged Class." *Advances in Alcohol and Substance Abuse* 4(2)(Winter 1984): 37-50.

Shore, Milton F. "Correlates and Concepts: Are We Chasing Our Tails?" *Etiology of Drug Abuse,* Research Monograph #56. Washington, DC: National Institute of Drug Abuse, 1985.

Smart, Reginald G. "Do Some Alcoholics Do Better In Some Types of Treatment Than Others?" *Drug and Alcohol Dependence* 3(1978): 65-75.

Smeeding, Timothy M. and Barbara Boyld Torrey. "Poor Children in Rich Countries." *Science* 243(1988): 873-77.

Smith, David. *A Multicultural View of Drug Abuse.* Cambridge MA: Schenkman, 1978.

Snyder, Charles B. *Alcohol and the Jews.* Glencoe: The Free Press, 1958.

Szasz, Thomas. Ceremonial Chemistry: *The Ritual Persecution of Drugs, Addicts and Pushers.* Garden City, NY: Anchor Press, 1974.

Taylor, Arnold. *American Diplomacy and Narcotics Traffic 1900-1939.* Durham, NC: Duke University Press, 1969.

Time. "Pop Goes the Bubble." 2 April 1990, 42.

——. "Our Bulging Prisons." 29 May 1989, 28-31.

——. "A Torrent of Dirty Dollars." 18 December 1989, 50-56.

——. "Panic Grips the Globe," 2 November 1987, 22-33.

——. "Wall Street's October Massacre." 26 October 1987, 32-33.

Toffler, Alvin. *The Third Wave.* New York: Morrow, 1980.

Trebach, Arnold. *The Great Drug War.* New York: Macmillan, 1987.

——. *The Heroin Solution.* New Haven: Yale University Press, 1982.

United Nations. *Monthly Bulletin of Statistics.* New York: Statistical Office of the United Nations. Vol. 43 (1) (1989): 96.

U.S. Bureau of the Census. *Statistical Abstract of the U.S. 1990.* #698. Washington, DC: U.S. Government Printing Office, 1990, 430.

——. *Statistical Abstract of the U.S. 1989.* #693. Washington, DC: U.S. Government Printing Office, 1989, 426.

——. *Statistical Abstract of the U.S. 1989.* #645. Washington, DC: U.S. Government Printing Office, 1989, 391.

——. *Statistical Abstract of the U.S. 1989.* #377. Washington, DC: U.S. Government Printing Office, 1989, 221.

United States Senate. *Drugs, Law Enforcement and Foreign Policy: A Report of the Subcommittee on Narcotics, Terrorism and International Operations,* Washington, DC: U.S. Government Printing Office, 1989.

Vaillant, George. *The Natural History of Alcoholism.* Cambridge, MA: Harvard University Press, 1985.

Veblen, Thorstein. *The Theory of the Leisure Class.* New York: Mentor, 1953 [1899].

Wallerstein, Immanuel. *The Modern World-System I: Capitalist Agriculture and the Origins of the European World Economy.* New York: Academic Press, 1974.

Watters, John K., Craig Reinarman, and Jeffrey Fagan. "Causality, Context and Contingency: Relationships Between Drug Abuse and Delinquency." *Contemporary Drug Problems* 12(3)(1985): 351-73.

Webster, Daniel W., Ernest Harburg, Lillian Gleiberman, Anthony

Schork, and Wayne Di Franceisco. "Familial Transmission of Alcohol Use I: Parent, and Adult Offspring Alcohol Use Over 17 Years—Tecumseh, Michigan." *Journal of Alcohol Studies* 50(6)(1989): 557-66.

Weismann, Adam Paul. "I was a Drug-Hype Junkie." *The New Republic*, 6 October 1986, 14-17.

Whyte, William Foote. *Street Corner Society*. Chicago: University of Chicago Press, 1943.

Willenbring, Mark L. "Measurement of Depression in Alcoholics." *Journal of Studies on Alcohol* 47(5)(1986):367-72.

Wilson, James Q. "Drugs and Crime." In *Drugs and Crime*, edited by James Q. Wilson and Michael Toney. Chicago: University of Chicago Press, 1990.

Wisotsky, Steven. *Breaking the Impasse in the War on Drugs*. New York: Greenwood Press, 1986.

Wisotsky, Steven. "Beyond the War on Drugs." In *The Drug Legalization Debate*, edited by James Inciardi. Newbury Park, CA: Sage Publications, 1991.

Witters, Weldon and Peter Venturelli. *Drugs and Society*. Boston: Jones and Bartlett, 1988.

Wolfgang, Marvin E. *Delinquency in a Birth Cohort*. Chicago: University of Chicago Press, 1972.

Zinn, Howard. *A People's History of the United States*. New York: Harper & Row, 1980.

Newspaper Articles

Christian Science Monitor
    6 November 1989. "Drug Crisis Burdens Prison System," 6:2.
    30 October 1989. "Cracking Down on Cargo Shippers," 7:2.

Daily Nexus
    2 June 1989. "Anti-Drug Statement Added For Pell Grant."

Los Angeles Times
    1 October 1991. "Aid For Indigent Addicts Failing, L.A. Study Finds,"A 1:4.
    7 September 1991. "Federal Judge Gets 6 Years in Bribe Plot," A 17:1.
    6 September 1991. "Doubts Cast on Crime Rates Ties to Drug War," A 20:1.
    2 July 1991. "Patriotism and Public Relations Paying Off for Escobar," H 3:1.
    20 June 1991. "3 Officers Acquitted in 39th-Dalton Raid," A 1:2.
    1 May 1991. "48% of Cancer Specialists in Study Would Prescribe Pot," A 12:1.
    29 March 1991. "$11.3 Million Paid in 1990 to Resolve Police Abuse Cases," A 3:1.
    23 March 1991. L.A. Officer Charged in Raid Pleads No Contest," B 1:1.

25 December 1990. "Middle Class Teens Copying Gangs," A 3:1.

28 June 1990. "Rose Wanted Part of Drug Ring, Janzen Says," D 1:1.

19 June 1990. "Drug Czar Assails State's Narcotics Laws as Too Weak," A 3:3.

7 June 1990. "Proposal Would Remove FBI as DEA Overseer," A 18:1.

1 June 1990. "Surgeon General Says Children Are Targets of Tobacco Industry," A 17:1.

23 May 1990. "Drug Cases Now Dominate Caseloads of Urban Courts," A 1:5.

22 May 1990. "Short Supplies May Be Diluting Street Cocaine," A 4:1.

21 May 1990. "Coca Price Collapse Offers Opportunity in Drug War," A 1:5.

21 May 1990. "Cocaine Related Deaths Decline for First Time in a Decade, Federal Figures Reveal," A 17:1.

21 May 1990 "California Leads U.S. in Inmate Increase," A 3:2.

16 May 1990. "Back Yard Brawl in Drug War," A 1:1.

6 May 1990. "Big Catch: Drug War's Little Fish," A 1:1.

23 April 1990. "Miami Trial Gives Startling New Portrait of Sam Gilbert," A 25:2.

22 April 1990. "Black Feel Brunt of Drug War," A 1:1.

18 April 1990. "Mexico to Confront U.S. on Camarena Case Abduction," A 1:5.

17 April 1990. "Under Fire: Women and Smoking," E 1:1.

6 April 1990. "Neglected Weapon in the Drug War," A 1:1.

12 March 1990 "Nothing Else Has Worked: Abolish the Prohibitions," B 7:1.

7 March 1990. "Bennett Scoffs at 'Touchy-Feely' Approach to Drug Prevention," A 15:1.

2 March 1990. "President Seeks to Reassure L.A. Deputy Sheriffs," A 1:5.

25 February 1990. "Mexico Pot Estimates Up Tenfold," A 1:6.

20 February 1990. "Crowded County Hospitals Suffer Crisis in Obstetrics," A 1:1.

18 February 1990. "Gold, Drugs and Clean Cash," *Los Angeles Times Magazine,* 10.

17 February 1990. "U.S. Ready to Admit World Cocaine Supplies are Vastly Underestimated," A 20:1.

15 February 1990. "Mother Turns in Son as Shooting Suspect," B 1:4.

6 February 1990. "U.S. Acts to Curb Exports of Drug-Making Solvents," A 1:5.

17 December 1989. "Bush Says He's Delighted by Death of Notorious Colombian Drug Lord," A 6:1.

17 December 1989. "Bloody Killing of Cocaine Kingpin Fills Colombia with Glee, Tension," A 7:1.

17 December 1989. "Ruling Backs U.S. Forces Police Role," A 1:4.

16 December 1989. "Colombian Police Kill Drug Lord," A 1:6.

16 December 1989. "Keystone Kops Drug Buy Near White House Mocked," A 30:1.

15 December 1989. "In Reversal, Military Seeks Drug War Role," A 1:4.

9 December 1989. "Kilroy Is There and Students Hope He'll Stay," A 1:1.

7 December 1989. "5 1/2 ounces of Crack Brings Life Term With No Parole," A 36:1.

5 December 1989. "Cocaine Has a Made in the U.S.A. Label," A1:1.

20 November 1989. "Drug Legalization:Interest Rises in Prestigious Circles," A 1:5.

15 November 1989. "Study Tightly Links Gangs to Trafficking in Cocaine," B 2:3.

14 November 1989. "Judges Probe Prosecutors Choices on Drug Arrests," B 1:5.

13 November 1989. "Schoolyard Drug Law Bias Charge to be Probed," B 1:5

6 November 1989. "5 Countries Freeze Drug Kingpins $60 Million," A 7:1.

6 November 1989. "Arrest Called Key Break in Sylmar Drug Bust Inquiry," A 1:3.

6 November 1989. "Federal Drug Prosecutions Lag in L.A," A 3:1.

6 November 1989. "The Science of Fighting a Drug War," A 1:1.

3 November 1989. "Key Suspect in Record Cocaine Haul is Captured," B 1:5.

23 October 1989. "Caribbean States Want U.N. in Drug War," A 5:3.

20 October 1989. "Don't Resist New Prisons, Bennett Pleads," A 22:1.

15 October 1989. "Colombia Extradites 3 to U.S.," A 1:6.

14 October 1989. "U.S. Okays Covert Operations That May Kill Foreigners," I 1:1.

6 October 1989. "9 Tons of Cocaine Seized in Texas," I 4:4.

5 October 1989. "Proposed Jail Seen as Symbol of Despair," II 1:1.

28 September 1989. "White House Calls Byrd Plan Price-Tag Politics," I 25:1.

27 September 1989. "Deputies Role Leads to Dismissal of Drug Case," I 1:1.

26 September 1989. "U.S. Seizes Property of Suspended Deputies," I 1:3.

24 September 1989. "Tiring of Fighting U.S. War,"

22 September 1989. "Drugs: Dutch Gain with Tolerant Tack," I 1:1.

19 September 1989. "Wider Anti-Drug Role Announced For Pentagon," I 6:1.

11 September 1989. "The Legacy of a Slaying," II 1:1.

10 September 1989. "Esther Crighton Has Respect: A 12-year old Fulfills His Mother's Dreams With Drug Profits," V 5:1.

8 September 1989. "Colombia Likely to Survive Loss of Drug Money," I 1:4.

7 September 1989. "Colombia Sends Drug Suspect to U.S. for Trial,"I 1:4.

7 September 1989. "Money Launderer of the Medallion Cartel Arrested," I 1:3.

6 September 1989. "Bush Tells Plan to Combat Drugs," I 1:5.

6 September 1989. "Plan Assailed as Not Aiding All Who Want Treatment," I 10:1.

2 September 1989. "Drug Funds Missing, 9 Deputies Suspended,"
I 1:2.

2 September 1989. "U.S. Probing Police Raid On Apartments," I 1:3.

30 August 1989. "Guatemala Seen Slipping Into a Haven For Drugs,"
I 1:2.

30 August 1989. "Tape Shows Israelis Training Cartel's Killers," I 1:2.

26 August 1989. "Officer Absolved Of Most Charges in Massive Raid,"
Ii 1:3.

18 August 1989. "Interagency Rivalries Said to Hinder Drug Fight,"
I 18:1.

4 August 1989. "U.S. Labels L.A. a Center of Drug Trade, Violence,"
I 1:4.

23 June 1989. "Lawyers Critical of Rulings on Seizure of Attorney
Fees," I 20:1.

14 June 1989. "Did Cocaine Sting Fuel Drug Sales," I 1:1.

14 June 1989. "South Lake Tahoe Mayor Accused in Drug, Money-
Laundering Case," I 3:1.

10 June 1989. "Mother Seized Under Gang Law Cleared," I 1:3.

31 May 1989. "Exclusionary Rule Appeal Refused by High Court,"
I 3:5.

31 May 1989. "Mother Arrested Under Gang Law Denies Blame," I 1:1.

12 May 1989. "U.S. Acts to Curb Exports of Drug-Making Solvents,"
I 21:1.

4 May 1989. "Bennett Outlines Anti-Drug Plan," I 1:5.

14 April 1989. "Ingenuity of Drug Lords on the Rise," I 1:1.

13 April 1989. "Cocaine Cuts New Routes to the North," I 1:1.

30 March 1989. "Cartel's Money Laundering Halted," I 12:1.

14 March 1989. "Angry Psychiatrists Denounce Threatened Mental
Health Cuts," I 3:1.

3 March 1989. "Bennett Would Limit Rights in War on Drugs," I 1:2.

24 February 1989. "Solid Gold Shock: Drug Money-Laundering Arrests
Stun Downtown Jewelry District," II 1:1.

1 December 1988. "Drug Cases Clog Justice System ABA Concludes,"
I 1:1.

28 November 1988. "Talent for the Drug Game: Tough and Loyal Athletes Recruited by Cocaine Rings," II 1:1.

23 November 1988. "3 Ex-U.S. Drug Agents Charged With IRS Fraud,"
II 1:5.

6 November 1988. "Seizures of Real Estate Stepped Up in War on
Drugs," I 1:1.

23 October 1988. "Police Departments Enjoy a Boom From Their Drug
Busts," II 1:4.

8 September 1988. "Black Gangs' Role in Drug Trade Overblown,
Study Finds," II 1:1.

24 August 1988. "Funds to Save Emergency Rooms Set," I 1:6.

10 August 1988. "Debate Resurrected Over Risks of Casual Drug Use,"
I 1:1.

17 May 1988. "Surgeon General Asserts Smoking is an Addiction,"
I 1:5.

11 January 1988. "Nofziger Resentful on Eve of Ethics Violation Trial," I 1:1.

18 November 1987. "Effectiveness of Roping Off Drug Areas Questioned," II 1:1.

New York Times

13 March 1990. "F.A.A. Faulted Over Crew That Drank," A 26:1.

6 February 1990. "Panama is Resisting U.S. Pressure to Alter Inadequate Bank Laws," A 1:1.

29 December 1989. "New Tactics in the War on Drugs Tilt Scales of Justice Off-Balance," I 1:1.

15 December 1989. "Intensive War on Drugs by Malaysia and Singapore Shows Mixed Results," I 12:1.

1 December 1989. "Budget Office Proposes $8 Billion Medicare Cut," I 26:4.

29 November 1989. "Reagan Proposes $7 Billion Cut in Health Payments," A 13:3.

27 November 1989. "Legalizing Drugs: Failures Spur Debate," A 9:4.

16 November 1989. "Emotionally Ill Pose Growing Burden to Police," A 1:2.

15 November 1989. "When Drugs and Despair Vie With 3Rs," I 1:2.

4 November 1989. "Colombia Judges and Their Aides Go On Strike to Demand Protection," A 4:1.

27 October 1989. "119 Seized in Drive to Halt Indoor Marijuana Growing," I 12:1.

20 October 1989. "Reality Intrudes on Drug Crusade in Capital," I 1:3.

19 September 1989. "In Making Drug Strategy, No Accord on Treatment," I 1:1.

21 August 1989. "Small Inner-City Hospitals in U.S. Face Threat of Financial Failure," I 1:4.

23 June 1989. "Depriving Drug Suspects of Lawyers Fees Ok'd," I 20:1.

2 March 1989. "Drug Production Rising Worldwide, State Dept. Says," I 1:3.

2 March 1989. "Children's Health Seen As Declining," I 21:1.

27 February 1989. "Treating Drug Addicts: Who Should Pay For It?" I 1:2.

30 January 1989. "Needle Plan Fails to Attract Drug Addicts So Its Revised," I 1:3.

11 January 1989. "U.S. Report Raises Estimate of Smoking Toll," I 20:4.

24 December 1988. "Cigarette Industry Financing Wide War on Smoking Bans," I 1:1.

27 November 1988. "Speed's Gain in Use could Rival Crack, Drug Experts Warn," I 1:1.

25 November 1988. "Armed, Sophisticated and Violent, Two Drug Gangs Blanket Nation," I 1:5.

27 September 1988. "Bush and Noriega: Examination of Their Ties," I 1:2.

9 September 1988. "House Votes Death fro Drug Murders," I 1:4.

9 September 1988. "Washington Talk," I 10:1.

28 August 1988. "Brazil Now a Vital Crossroad for Latin Cocaine Traffickers," I 1:1.

23 June 1988. "Addiction's Hidden Toll: Poor Families in Turmoil," I 1:1.

8 May 1988. "Officials Say Bush Heard '85 Charge Against Noriega," I 1:3.

2 May 1988. "Young Crack Addicts Find There's No Help For Them," II 1:2.

10 April 1988. "Fighting Narcotics: U.S. is Urged to Shift Tactics," I 1:1.

31 January 1988. "Addicts to Get Needles in Plan to Curb AIDS," I 1:1.

22 January 1988. "Crime Study Finds Recent Drug Use in Most Arrested," I 1:6.

Santa Barbara Independent

8 September 1988. "Reaching Out: The Rape Crisis Center Fights for Lives."

Santa Barbara News-Press

29 August 1989. "Probation Demand Tough For Addicts."

12 January 1989. "N.Y. Study Links Cocaine to Road Deaths."

Wall Street Journal

7 September 1989. Milton Friedman, "An Open Letter to Bill Bennett," A 14:3.

17 January 1989. "Cocaine Rebellion: Peru's Guerrillas Draw Support of Peasants in Coca-Rich Regions," A 1:1.

25 November 1986. "Many Mexican Police Supplement Low Pay with Tips and Fines," A 1:4.

19 November 1986. "Death of U.S. Agent in Mexico Drug Case Uncovers Grid of Graft," A 1:1.

The Washington Post

16 December 1989. "U.S. Anti-Drug Effort Called Wrong for DC," A 1:4.

13 December 1989. "U.S. Judge Calls for Legalization of Illicit Drugs," A 1:1.

Index

The Medicine Society

Production Editor: Martha Bates
Cover Design: Sean T. Harrington
Cover Photography: Michael Smith

Text composed by Michael J. Brooks in $^{10}/_{11.5}$ Melior

Printed by Bookcrafters on 60# Lakewood